FAMILY GUIDE TO

Prescription Drugs

THE AUTHOR

Dorothy L. Smith, Pharm. D.

Director of Clinical Affairs,
American Pharmaceutical Assoc.

THE REVIEW COMMITTEE

Thomas A. Gossel, R.Ph., PH.D.
Henry A. Palmer, Ph.D.
Nicholas G. Popovich, Ph.D.
J. Richard Wuest, Pharm. D., R.Ph.

published by:

A division of
Automatic Business Products, Co., Inc.
Tuckie Road, P.O. Box 57
Willimantic, CT 06226

First Printing, September, 1980
Second Printing, February, 1981

Printed in the U.S.A.

Table of Contents

3

PREFACE

Whenever a doctor prescribes a medication for a patient, he carefully selects a drug which he feels will be of the most benefit. He expects the patient to take the prescription to a pharmacy and to follow the prescription instructions. However, it has been shown that approximately 50% of all patients make medication errors. Drugs taken incorrectly can either be less effective or, even worse, medically harmful.

In order for a drug to be effective, it must be properly prescribed by the doctor, properly dispensed by the pharmacist and ACCURATELY ADMINISTERED BY THE PATIENT. For several years, I have been concerned with the high number of errors patients make when they are taking prescription drugs. One of the most common reasons for these errors is a lack of knowledge. The directions on a prescription label are almost always incomplete and do not provide enough information for a person who is responsible for treating himself or a family member. "Take 1 capsule every 6 hours" or "Take as directed" are inadequate instructions. Some of the medications in order to be most effective require special methods of administration and should not be taken with certain kinds of food. For example, the antibiotic tetracycline should not be taken with milk or dairy products and penicillin G should not be taken at mealtime. Many drugs can interact with each other and should not be taken at the same time. Alcoholic beverages should also be avoided while some medications are being taken. There are some medications which commonly cause minor side effects. For example, if a tranquilizer causes drowsiness during the first few days of treatment, care should be taken to avoid driving a car or doing dangerous jobs during this time. People taking prescription drugs have to trust the judgments and skills of their doctors and pharmacists. However, it is also important that they be informed of the basic medication instructions in order to help receive maximum benefit from the treatment.

The medication instructions contained in this book have been prepared in cooperation with several leading physicians and pharmacists in the United States and Canada. They were originally prepared as individual leaflets for patients and then as a binder to be used by pharmacists. In response to requests from health care professionals and patients, the medication instructions have been printed in this form with the hope that they will reinforce the verbal instructions of the physician and pharmacist and can be referred to by the patient at a later date. Instructions have been prepared for the most commonly prescribed medications and the basic text for each drug consists of the following information:

1. USUAL PURPOSE (S) OF THE MEDICINE
2. CORRECT METHOD OF ADMINISTRATION
3. CORRECT TIMES OF ADMINISTRATION
4. COMMON SIDE EFFECTS AND APPROPRIATE PRECAUTIONS
5. WHEN THE PHYSICIAN SHOULD BE CONSULTED
6. DRUG INTERACTIONS WITH FOOD, ALCOHOL AND NON-PRESCRIPTION MEDICINES
7. SPECIAL STORAGE REQUIREMENTS

It cannot be emphasized too greatly that these medication instructions are general in nature and are to be used only under the direction and guidance of a health care professional.

Be sure to carefully read **How to Use Your Medicines Safely.** This special section contains information that applies to the safe use of any medicine. Do not become alarmed if the instructions are slightly altered by your doctor or pharmacist. It is only because of your other drug therapy or medical conditions that the instructions will be altered to suit you personally. It is extremely important to tell your doctor and pharmacist if you are pregnant, plan to become pregnant, breast-feeding, allergic to any drugs or if you have a kidney or liver disease.

The medications a person is presently taking or has taken in the past could be very important to any future drugs his physician or dentist may prescribe. It is extremely important that you have all your prescriptions filled at the SAME pharmacy especially if you are being treated by more than one doctor. Just as your physician keeps your medical record, many pharmacists keep drug records or profiles for their patients. The pharmacist who knows your complete medication history is in a better position to assist your doctors, as well as to advise you about nonprescription drugs which you can safely use.

Two PERSONAL MEDICATION RECORD cards are included in this book and it is recommended that you and your family members complete them and carry them in your wallets. This personal drug record could be valuable if you are ever in an accident. The doctors treating you would know immediately what allergies you may have and which drugs you have been taking. The record card could even help save your life!

Every person who receives a prescription for a medication has a very important role to play in his drug treatment. Only if the medication is CORRECTLY taken can one expect to receive the most benefit. Otherwise, the drug treatment will be a failure. I hope that the medication instructions in this book will help you to remember the verbal instructions you receive from your doctor or pharmacist.

February, 1981   **Dorothy L. Smith, B.S.P., Pharm.D.**

ABOUT THE AUTHOR

Dr. Smith has devoted most of her professional life to the improvement of patient education. Her experience includes nine years of teaching in U.S. and Canadian Colleges of Pharmacy and five years as Coordinator of Ambulatory Pharmacy Care at Toronto's Sunnybrook Medical Center. This background has given her a unique insight into the communication needs of both patients and health care professionals.

She is the editor of the Lea and Febiger textbook **Medication Guide for Patient Counseling** and the Pharmex publications **Patient Advisory Leaflets** and **Consumer's Guide to Prescription Product Information.** Her expertise has influenced pharmacy educators and students as well as doctors, pharmacists and nurses throughout North America.

PUBLISHER'S NOTE

The information presented in **Prescription Drugs** is not intended to represent all the available information on the medications presented. Considerable care has been taken to ensure the accuracy of the information contained herein. The editor and publisher cannot be responsible for errors in publication or any consequences arising from the use of the information contained in this book.

If you have **ANY** questions regarding the drug you are taking, always ask your pharmacist or doctor.

How to Use Your Medicines Safely

Prescription Medicine

1. Not all medical conditions require the use of medications. You doctor has carefully prescribed your medicines for you because he believes that they are the best possible treatment for your particular condition. In order for you to receive the greatest benefit from you drugs, it is essential that you take them **exactly** as your doctor has prescribed. This information is on the prescription label – **be sure to read the label carefully.** If you should have any questions about your medications which the label does not answer, ask your pharmacist or your doctor.

2. Whenever you receive a medication from a pharmacist, YOU SHOULD KNOW THE ANSWER TO THESE QUESTIONS:

What is the name of the medication?
What is the purpose of the medication?
Are there any precautions you should be aware of while you are taking the medication?
Are there any other medications you should not take at the same time?
Is there any food or beverage you should avoid?
How and when should you take the medication?
How long should you continue to take the medication?
Can the prescription be refilled and how?

3. Have all your prescriptions filled at the same pharmacy so that the pharmacist can keep a complete record of your medicines Do not go without medicine between prescription refills. Call you pharmacist 1 or 2 days before you will need the repeat of you prescription.

4. If you visit more than one doctor, tell each one what medicines you are taking. This should include prescription and nonprescription drugs as both could interfere with a new medication that the doctor may prescribe for you. Always tell your doctor if you did not have a prescription filled or if you did not take your medication. Otherwise, he may conclude that the medication was not effective. It is important that you take the medication your doctor has prescribed for you; only by taking it will you derive any benefit from your medication.

5. In addition to their benefits, most drugs have additional minor actions. These are called side effects and are usually not detrimental to your health. You may not experience any side effects from a drug. Side effects vary from one patient to another, and at times a particular medication produces an unpleasant side effect in one patient, whereas another medication that is almost identical will have no unpleasant effect. If you think your medicine is causing a problem, call your doctor or pharmacist and let him know. He can tell you if the problem is due to the medicine and can make any necessary adjustments.

Allergies
6. Always tell your doctor and pharmacist if you are allergic to any drugs or other substances or if you have had any unpleasant reactions to drugs. Call your doctor immediately if you think you may be allergic to a medicine or if you develop a skin rash, itching, hives, swelling of the face or difficulty in breathing.

7. Remember that the medicine you have received is specifically for you. DO NOT SHARE it with other members of your family or your friends who seem to have the same symptoms you have. They should see their own doctor who will decide which is the best treatment for them.

Nonprescription Medicines
8. Be careful in treating yourself with **any medication you can purchase without a prescription (for example, aspirin, laxatives, vitamins, cough medicines).** Always read the directions on the folder and if you do not understand them, consult your pharmacist. These medicines are usually designed to alleviate a symptom and they do not cure a disease. Do not continue using the medicine if the first few doses do not help to relieve the symptom. If a symptom is severe or persistent, check with your doctor.

9. If you are taking a drug that has been prescribed by your physician, always be careful in self-medicating with drugs you can purchase without a prescription, i.e., cough syrups, laxatives, nasal sprays. Some drugs can interact and cause unpleasant reactions. Always check with your pharmacist before you purchase these products.

Pregnancy & Breast-Feeding
10. Women who are **pregnant** or **breast-feeding** or **plan to become pregnant** should not take any medications or home remedies without consulting their doctor or pharmacist.

Children
11. Do not give any medicine to a **child** less than one year of age unless it has been prescribed by your doctor. Do not give any no prescription drugs to children between 1 and 12 years of age u less the doses for the different age groups are listed on the packa container.

Storage of Medicines
12. The way in which you store your drugs is important. Certa drugs require refrigeration. If this is the case, there will be a **Ke Refrigerated** label on the container. Do not store **ANY** medicin in the refrigerator unless specified by your pharmacist. A cool, c dark cupboard is the best storage place for most other medication Remember that your bathroom medicine cupboard often becomes I and steamy and is not the best place to store your medicatio Above all, keep your medicines in a safe place and away from I reach and sight of small children.

13. Always keep your medicine in the container in which you receiv it from the pharmacist. Do NOT remove the label until all the me ication is finished. The information on the label is necessary properly identify the patient, the physician, the drug, the instructio for use, and the date the prescription was dispensed.

14. Over the years you may have had numerous drugs prescrib for you. If these drugs are discontinued by your doctor, destr the remaining portion by flushing it down the toilet. By doing t you avoid building up a cupboard of old, outdated, and potentia dangerous drugs.

Personal Medication Record Card
15. It is recommended that you carry a card in your wallet t lists important facts about your health and your medications. T allows you to have a complete list of your medications if you sho see another doctor. If you move to another neighborhood, you sho carefully choose your new pharmacy and doctor. It is important t your new pharmacist and doctor are thoroughly familiar with t medicines you are taking and your medical history.

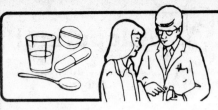

Acetaminophen-Codeine

Common Trade Names:
**Phenaphen with Codeine,
Tylenol with Codeine**

 This medicine is used to help relieve pain.

Do not take this medicine more often or longer than your doctor has prescribed.

 In some people this drug may cause dizziness or drowsiness. Do not drive a car or operate dangerous machinery or do jobs that require you to be alert until you know how you are going to react to this drug. If you become dizzy, you should be careful going up and down stairs. Sit or lie down at the first sign of dizziness.

 Do not drink alcoholic beverages while taking this drug.

 It is important that you obtain the advice of your doctor before taking other pain relievers, non-prescription drugs, sleeping pills or tranquilizers while you are taking this drug.

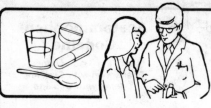

Allopurinol

Common Trade Names:
Zyloprim

This medicine is used to treat gout and other diseases in which the body has high levels of uric acid.

Take this medicine with food or after meals.

It is important that you take this medicine as your doctor has prescribed and try not to miss any doses. Do not stop taking the medicine without consulting your doctor.

In some people, this drug may cause drowsiness. Do not drive a car or operate dangerous machinery or do jobs that require you to be alert until you know how you are going to react to this drug.

It is recommended that you try to drink at least 8 to 10 glasses of water or other liquids every day while you are taking this medicine.

Call your doctor if you develop a skin rash.

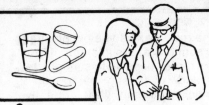

Amitriptyline
Elavil
Imipramine
Tofranil

 This medicine is used to help relieve the symptoms of depression and has been used in children to treat bed-wetting.

 The full effect of this medicine will not be noticed immediately but may take from a few days to 4 weeks.

 In some people, this drug may cause dizziness or drowsiness. Do not drive a car or operate dangerous machinery or do jobs that require you to be alert until you know how you are going to react to this drug.

 If this medicine causes dizziness, you should be careful going up and down stairs and you should not change positions too rapidly. Get out of bed slowly in the morning and dangle your feet over the edge of the bed for a few minutes before standing. Sit or lie down at the first sign of dizziness. Tell your doctor you have been dizzy.

 Do not drink alcoholic beverages while taking this drug.

It is important that you obtain the advice of your doctor before taking pain relievers, nonprescription drugs, sleeping pills or tranquilizers while you are taking this drug.

 Suck a hard sour candy (sugarless), ice chips or chew gum if your mouth becomes dry. It is especially important to brush your teeth regularly if you develop a dry mouth.

This medicine may make some people more sensitive to sunlight and sunlamps. If your skin becomes more sensitive to sunlight, tell your doctor and try to stay out of direct sunlight. While in the sun, wear protective clothing and sunglasses. You may wish to ask your pharmacist about suitable sunscreen products. Call your doctor if you become sunburned.

Do not stop taking this medicine suddenly without the approval of your doctor.

Call your doctor if you develop a sore throat, fever, mouth sores, eye pain, or difficulty in urinating (passing your water).

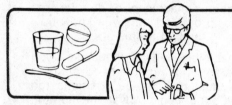

Amitriptyline-Perphenazine

Common Trade Names:
Etrafon, Triavil

This medicine is used to help relieve the symptoms of anxiety and depression.

The full effect of this medicine will not be noticed immediately but may take from a few days to 4 weeks.

In some people, this drug may cause dizziness or drowsiness. Do not drive a car or operate dangerous machinery or do jobs that require you to be alert until you know how you are going to react to this drug.

If this medicine causes dizziness, you should be careful going up and down stairs and you should not change positions too rapidly. Get out of bed slowly in the morning and dangle your feet over the edge of the bed for a few minutes before standing. Sit or lie down at the first sign of dizziness. Tell your doctor you have been dizzy.

Do not drink alcoholic beverages while taking this drug.

It is important that you obtain the advice of your doctor before taking pain relievers, non-prescription drugs, sleeping pills or tranquilizers while you are taking this drug.

Suck a hard sour candy (sugarless), ice chips or chew gum if your mouth becomes dry. It is especially important to brush your teeth regularly if you develop a dry mouth.

This medicine may make some people more sensitive to sunlight or sunlamps. If your skin becomes more sensitive to sunlight, tell your doctor and try to stay out of direct sunlight. While in the sun, wear protective clothing and sunglasses. You may wish to ask your pharmacist about suitable sunscreen products. Call your doctor if you become sunburned.

Do not stop taking this medicine suddenly without the approval of your doctor.

Call your doctor if you develop a sore throat, fever, mouth sores, eye pain, difficulty in urinating (passing your water), dark-colored urine, a yellow color in the eyes or skin, or unusual movements of the face, tongue or arms.

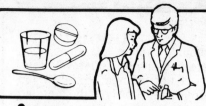

Amoxicillin

Common Trade Names:
Amoxil, Larotid

 This medicine is an antibiotic used to treat certain types of infections.

This medicine may be taken with meals or on an empty stomach.

 For Liquid Medicines:
• Store the bottle of medicine in the refrigerator but do not freeze.

 • Each time you use it, shake the bottle well so that you can measure an accurate dose.

 • If a dropper is used to measure the dose and you do not fully understand how to use it, check with your pharmacist.

 • If there is a discard date on the bottle, throw away any unused medicine after that date. Do not take or save old medicine. Call your pharmacist if you are not sure of the discard date.

 It is important to take **all** of this medicine plus any refills that your doctor told you to take. Do not stop taking it earlier than your doctor has recommended in spite of the fact that you may feel better. Otherwise, the infection may return.

 This medicine sometimes causes diarrhea (loose bowel movements). Call your doctor if the diarrhea becomes severe or lasts for more than two days.

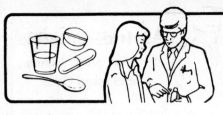

Ampicillin

Common Trade Names:
Amcill, Omnipen, Penbritin, Polycillin, Principen

This medicine is an antibiotic used to treat certain types of infections.

This medicine should be taken on an empty stomach at least 1 hour before (or 2 hours after) food unless otherwise directed. Take it at the proper time even if you skip a meal.

For Liquid Medicines:

Store the bottle of medicine in a refrigerator but do not freeze.

Each time you use it, shake the bottle well so that you can measure an accurate dose.

If a dropper is used to measure the dose and you do not fully understand how to use it, check with your pharmacist.

If there is a discard date on the bottle, throw away any unused medicine after that date. Do not take or save old medicine. Call your pharmacist if you are not sure of the discard date.

It is important to take **all** of this medicine plus any refills that your doctor told you to take. Do not stop taking it earlier than your doctor has recommended in spite of the fact that you may feel better. Otherwise, the infection may return.

This medicine sometimes causes diarrhea (loose bowel movements). Call your doctor if the diarrhea becomes severe or lasts for more than two days.

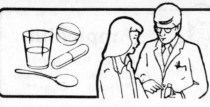

Aspirin - Codeine

Common Trade Names:

Empirin with Codeine

This medicine is used to help relieve pain and fever.

Do not take this medicine more often or longer than your doctor has prescribed.

It is best to take this medicine with a glass of milk or food to help prevent stomach upset. Call your doctor if you continue to have stomach upset.

In some people this drug may cause dizziness or drowsiness. Do not drive a car or operate dangerous machinery or do jobs that require you to be alert until you know how you are going to react to this drug. If you become dizzy, you should be careful going up and down stairs. Sit or lie down at the first sign of dizziness.

Do not drink alcoholic beverages while taking this drug.

It is important that you obtain the advice of your doctor before taking other pain relievers, non-prescription drugs, sleeping pills or tranquilizers while you are taking this drug.

Call your doctor if you develop "ringing" or "buzzing" in the ears or difficulty hearing, black stools, fever, sweating, wheezing or unusual fatigue or nervousness.

Do not take or save old medicine. Throw away this medicine if it smells like vinegar.

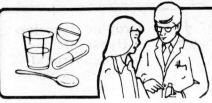

APC-Oxycodone

Common Trade Names:
Percodan

 This medicine is used to help relieve pain.

Do not take this medicine more often or longer than your doctor has prescribed.

 It is best to take this medicine with a glass of milk or food to help prevent stomach upset. Call your doctor if you continue to have stomach upset.

 In some people this drug may cause dizziness or drowsiness. Do not drive a car or operate dangerous machinery or do jobs that require you to be alert until you know how you are going to react to this drug. If you become dizzy, you should be careful going up and down stairs. Sit or lie down at the first sign of dizziness.

 Do not drink alcoholic beverages while taking this drug.

 It is important that you obtain the advice of your doctor before taking other pain relievers, non-prescription drugs, sleeping pills or tranquilizers while you are taking this drug.

 Call your doctor if you develop "ringing" or "buzzing" in the ears or difficulty hearing, black stools, fever, sweating, difficulty in breathing, or unusual fatigue or nervousness. Your doctor should also know if you develop constipation or have difficulty urinating (passing your water).

 Do not take or save old medicine. Throw away this medicine if it smells like vinegar.

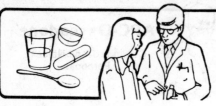

This medicine is used to help decrease stomach secretions and relax stomach and bowel muscles.

Suck a hard sour candy (sugarless), ice chips or chew gum if your mouth becomes dry. It is especially important to brush your teeth regularly if you develop a dry mouth.

In some people, this drug may cause drowsiness or blurred vision. Do not drive a car or operate dangerous machinery or do jobs that require you to be alert until you know how you are going to react to this drug.

A desire to urinate (passing your water) with an inability to do so is a side effect that may occur with this drug. Urinating at the time of taking the drug may help to relieve this problem. Tell your doctor if you are having this problem.

Do not drink alcoholic beverages while taking this drug.

It is important that you obtain the advice of your doctor before taking pain relievers, nonprescription drugs, sleeping pills or tranquilizers while you are taking this drug.

Do not take this medicine more often or longer than prescribed by your doctor.

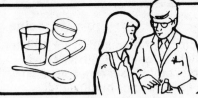

Betamethasone Valerate

Common Trade Names:
Valisone

This medicine is used to help relieve pain, itching, redness and swelling of certain types of skin conditions.

Instructions for use:

If you were prescribed the CREAM or OINTMENT:

• Cleanse the skin area well with soap and water unless otherwise directed by your doctor. Allow the skin to dry completely or pat dry with a clean towel.

• Apply the drug to the affected area and rub in lightly. Do not bandage unless directed by your doctor.

If you were prescribed the SPRAY:

• Cleanse the skin well with soap and water unless otherwise directed by your doctor. Allow the skin to dry completely or pat dry with a clean towel.

• Spray the affected area from about 6 inches away and do not spray for more than 3 seconds.

• Do not inhale the spray.

• Do not place the container in hot water or near radiators, stoves or other sources of heat. Store in a cool place. Do not puncture or burn the container (even when it is empty).

Do not use the drug more frequently or in larger quantities than prescribed by your doctor.

Do not apply cosmetics or lotions on top of the drug unless your doctor approves.

Call your doctor if the condition for which this medication is being used persists or becomes worse, or if it causes a constant irritation such as itching or burning.

For external use only. Keep this drug away from the eyes.

Brompheniramine
Dimetane

Brompheniramine-
Phenylephrine-
Phenylpropanolamine
Dimetapp

Brompheniramine-
Phenylephrine-
Phenylpropanolamine-
Guaifenesin-
Dimetane Expectorant

Brompheniramine- Phenylephrine-
Phenylpropanolamine- Guaifenesin-Codeine
Dimetane Expectorant-DC

This medicine is used to help relieve the symptoms of certain types of allergic conditions, coughs and colds, and certain skin conditions.

This drug may be taken with food if it upsets your stomach.

If you were prescribed EXTENTABS, swallow the medicine whole. Do not chew, crush or break it into pieces.

In some people this drug may cause dizziness or drowsiness. Do not drive a car or operate dangerous machinery or do jobs that require you to be alert until you know how you are going to react to this drug. If you become dizzy, you should be careful going up and down stairs. Sit or lie down at the first sign of dizziness.

Do not drink alcoholic beverages while taking this drug.

It is important that you obtain the advice of your doctor before taking pain relievers, nonprescription drugs, sleeping pills or tranquilizers while you are taking this drug.

Do not use this medicine more often or longer than recommended by your doctor.

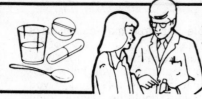

Butabarbital

Common Trade Names:
Buticaps, Butisol Sodium

This medicine is used as a sleeping pill and for certain kinds of nervousness.

In some people, this drug may cause dizziness or drowsiness. Do not drive a car or operate dangerous machinery or do jobs that require you to be alert until you know how you are going to react to this drug.

If you become dizzy, you should be careful going up and down stairs. Sit or lie down at the first sign of dizziness.

Do not drink alcoholic beverages while taking this drug.

It is important that you obtain the advice of your doctor before taking pain relievers, nonprescription drugs, sleeping pills or tranquilizers while you are taking this drug.

Do not take any more of this drug than your doctor has prescribed and do not stop taking it suddenly without first asking your doctor.

If you are taking this medicine to help you sleep, go to bed after you have taken it. Do not smoke in bed after you have taken it and do not store this medicine at your bedside.

Call your doctor if you develop bothersome sleepiness or laziness during the day, nightmares, staggering or unusual nervousness.

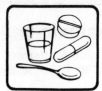

Butalbital-APC
Common Trade Names:
Fiorinal

Butalbital-APC-Codeine
Common Trade Names:
Fiorinal with Codeine

This medicine is used to help relieve pain and tension.

Do not take the medicine more often or longer than your doctor has prescribed.

It is best to take this medicine with food or a glass of water to help prevent stomach upset. Call your doctor if you continue to have stomach upset.

In some people this drug may cause dizziness or drowsiness. Do not drive a car or operate dangerous machinery or do jobs that require you to be alert until you know how you are going to react to this drug. If you become dizzy, you should be careful going up and down stairs. Sit or lie down at the first sign of dizziness.

Do not drink alcoholic beverages while taking this drug.

It is important that you obtain the advice of your doctor before taking other pain relievers, non-prescription drugs, sleeping pills or tranquilizers while you are taking this drug.

Call your doctor if you develop "ringing" or "buzzing" in the ears or difficulty hearing, black stools, fever, sweating, wheezing or unusual fatigue or nervousness.

Do not take or save old medicine. Throw away this medicine if it smells like vinegar.

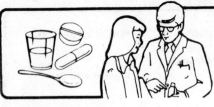

Cephalexin

Common Trade Names:
Keflex

This medicine is an antibiotic used to treat certain types of infections.

It is best to take this medicine on an empty stomach at least 1 hour before (or 2 hours after) eating food. Take it at the proper time even if you skip a meal. If you develop an upset stomach after taking the drug, take it with some food. Call your doctor if you continue to have an upset stomach.

For Liquid Medicines:

Store the bottle of medicine in a refrigerator but do not freeze.

Each time you use it, shake the bottle well so that you can measure an accurate dose.

If a dropper is used to measure the dose and you do not fully understand how to use it, check with your pharmacist.

If there is a discard date on the bottle, throw away any unused medicine after that date. Do not take or save old medicine. Call your pharmacist if you are not sure of the discard date.

It is important to take **all** of this medicine plus any refills that your doctor told you to take. Do not stop taking it earlier than your doctor has recommended in spite of the fact that you may feel better. Otherwise, the infection may return.

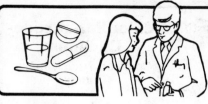

Chlordiazepoxide

Common Trade Names:
Librium

This medicine is used to help relieve anxiety and tension. It is also used to help relax muscles and to treat some conditions of the nerves.

In some people, this drug may cause dizziness or drowsiness. Do not drive a car or operate dangerous machinery or do jobs that require you to be alert until you know how you are going to react to this drug.

If you become dizzy, you should be careful going up and down stairs. Sit or lie down at the first sign of dizziness.

Do not drink alcoholic beverages while taking this drug.

It is important that you obtain the advice of your doctor before taking pain relievers, nonprescription drugs, sleeping pills or tranquilizers while you are taking this drug.

Do not stop taking this medicine suddenly without the advice of your doctor.

Call your doctor if you develop a sore throat, fever, mouth sores, extreme fatigue, fast heart beats, or staggering.

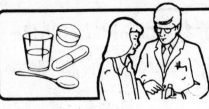

Chlordiazepoxide-Clidinium

Common Trade Names:
Librax

 This medicine is used to treat stomach and bowel conditions.

 In some people, this drug may cause dizziness or drowsiness. Do not drive a car or operate dangerous machinery or do jobs that require you to be alert until you know how you are going to react to this drug.

 If you become dizzy, you should be careful going up and down stairs. Sit or lie down at the first sign of dizziness.

 Do not drink alcoholic beverages while taking this drug.

 It is important that you obtain the advice of your doctor before taking pain relievers, nonprescription drugs, sleeping pills or tranquilizers while you are taking this drug.

Do not stop taking this medicine suddenly without the advice of your doctor.

 Suck a hard sour candy (sugarless), ice chips or chew gum if your mouth becomes dry. It is especially important to brush your teeth regularly if you develop a dry mouth.

 Call your doctor if you develop a sore throat, fever, mouth sores, extreme fatigue, staggering, fast heart beats or blurred vision.

Chlorpheniramine
Chlor-Trimeton, Teldrin

Chlorpheniramine-Phenylpropanolamine
Ornade

Chlorpheniramine-Isopropamide-Phenylpropanolamine-Caramiphen
Tuss-Ornade

Chlorpheniramine- Phenylpropanolamine-Phenylephrine- Phenyltoloxamine

Naldecon

 This medicine is used to help relieve the symptoms of colds and certain types of allergic conditions.

This drug may be taken with food if it upsets your stomach.

 If you were prescribed EXTENTABS, SPANSULES or NALDECON TABLETS, swallow the medicine whole. Do not crush, chew or break it into pieces.

 If NALDECON PEDIATRIC DROPS were prescribed, use the special dropper that comes with the medicine. If you have any questions about how to use it, ask your pharmacist.

 In some people, this drug may cause dizziness or drowsiness. Do not drive a car or operate dangerous machinery or do jobs that require you to be alert until you know how you are going to react to this drug.

 If you become dizzy, you should be careful going up and down stairs. Sit or lie down at the first sign of dizziness.

 Do not drink alcoholic beverages while taking this drug.

It is important that you obtain the advice of your doctor before taking pain relievers, nonprescription drugs, sleeping pills or tranquilizers while you are taking this drug.

Suck a hard sour candy (sugarless), ice chips or chew gum if your mouth becomes dry. It is especially important to brush your teeth regularly if you develop a dry mouth.

Call your doctor if you develop blurred vision, weakness, or troublesome drowsiness.

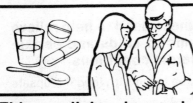

Chlorpromazine

Common Trade Names:
Thorazine

This medicine is used to help relieve the symptoms of anxiety and tension and certain types of emotional problems. This drug has several other uses and the reason it was prescribed depends upon your condition. Check with your doctor if you do not fully understand why you are taking it.

If you were prescribed THORAZINE SPANSULES, swallow the capsules whole. Do not crush, chew or mash the contents.

If you were prescribed SUPPOSITORIES:

● Remove the wrapper from the suppository.

● Lie on your side and raise your knee to your chest.

● Insert the suppository with the tapered (pointed) end first into the rectum. Hold the suppository in place for a few minutes.

● Try to avoid having a bowel movement for at least one hour so that the drug can be absorbed.

In some people, this drug may cause dizziness or drowsiness. Do not drive a car or operate dangerous machinery or do jobs that require you to be alert until you know how you are going to react to this drug.

Do not drink alcoholic beverages while taking this drug.

It is important that you obtain the advice of your doctor before taking pain relievers, non-prescription drugs, sleeping pills or tranquilizers while you are taking this drug.

This medicine makes some people more sensitive to sunlight or sunlamps. If your skin becomes more sensitive to sunlight, tell your doctor and try to stay out of direct sunlight. While in the sun, wear protective clothing and sunglasses. You may wish to ask your pharmacist about suitable sunscreen products. Call your doctor if you become sunburned.

If this medicine causes dizziness, you should be careful going up and down stairs and you should not change positions too rapidly. Get out of bed slowly in the morning and dangle your feet over the edge of the bed for a few minutes before standing up. Sit or lie down at the first sign of dizziness. Tell your doctor you have been dizzy.

Suck a hard sour candy (sugarless), ice chips or chew gum if your mouth becomes dry. It is especially important to brush your teeth regularly if you develop a dry mouth.

Do not stop taking this medicine suddenly without the approval of your doctor.

Call your doctor if you develop a sore throat, fever, mouth sores, skin rash, changes in eyesight, dark-colored urine, a yellow color in the eyes or skin, or unusual movements of the face, tongue or arms.

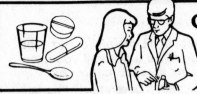

Chlorpropamide

Common Trade Names:
Diabinese

This medicine is used in the treatment of diabetes.

Take the drug with food if it upsets your stomach. Call your doctor if you continue to have stomach upset.

Know the signs of hypoglycemia (low blood sugar). Call your doctor if you develop weakness, sweating or shaking that is not relieved by eating or drinking something sweet.

It is very important that you take this drug as your doctor has prescribed and that you do not miss any doses. Take this medicine at the same time every day and do not go without this medicine between prescription refills.

It is recommended that patients avoid the use of alcoholic beverages because the combination may cause headache, flushing or an upset stomach.

Your doctor or pharmacist can tell you which nonprescription medicines (for example, cough medicines) are safe for diabetic patients.

Call your doctor if you develop a sore throat, fever, mouth sores, diarrhea (loose bowel movements), dark-colored urine, light-colored stools, or a yellow color in the eyes or skin.

Carry a card in your wallet or wear a bracelet stating that you are a diabetic.

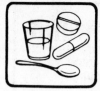

Chlorzoxazone-Acetaminophen

Common Trade Names:
Parafon Forte

 This medicine is used to help relieve muscle pain and stiffness.

 In some people, this drug may cause dizziness or drowsiness. Do not drive a car or operate dangerous machinery or do jobs that require you to be alert until you know how you are going to react to this drug.

 If you become dizzy, you should be careful going up and down stairs. Sit or lie down at the first sign of dizziness.

Do not take this medicine more often or longer than your doctor has prescribed.

 Do not drink alcoholic beverages while taking this drug.

 It is important that you obtain the advice of your doctor before taking pain relievers, non-prescription drugs, sleeping pills or tranquilizers while you are taking this drug.

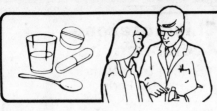

Cimetidine

Common Trade Names
Tagamet

This medicine is used in the treatment of certain types of stomach conditions.

Take this medicine with food or immediately after meals unless otherwise directed.

In some people, this drug may cause dizziness. Do not drive a car or operate dangerous machinery or do jobs that require you to be alert until you know how you are going to react to this drug. Sit or lie down at the first sign of dizziness.

Be sure to take this medicine exactly as directed by your doctor. Do not miss any doses.

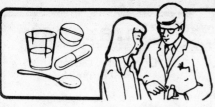

Clofibrate

Common Trade Names:
Atromid-S

This medicine is used in certain types of conditions to lower the amount of cholesterol and triglycerides (fatty substances) in the blood.

Take this medicine with food or immediately after meals to help prevent stomach upset.

In some people, this drug may cause dizziness or drowsiness. Do not drive a car or operate dangerous machinery or do jobs that require you to be alert until you know how you are going to react to this drug.

If you become dizzy, you should be careful going up and down stairs. Sit or lie down at the first sign of dizziness.

It is very important to follow any diet that your doctor may also prescribe for you.

Call your doctor if you develop a skin rash, nausea or vomiting, sore or aching muscles, muscle cramps or swelling of the legs or ankles.

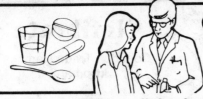

Clorazepate

Common Trade Names:
Tranxene

This medicine is used to help relieve anxiety and to treat some conditions of the nerves.

If you were prescribed TRANXENE-SD, swallow the tablets whole. Do not crush, chew or break them into pieces.

In some people, this drug may cause dizziness or drowsiness. Do not drive a car or operate dangerous machinery or do jobs that require you to be alert until you know how you are going to react to this drug.

If you become dizzy, you should be careful going up and down stairs. Sit or lie down at the first sign of dizziness.

Do not drink alcoholic beverages while taking this drug.

It is important that you obtain the advice of your doctor before taking pain relievers, non-prescription drugs, sleeping pills or tranquilizers while you are taking this drug.

Suck a hard sour candy (sugarless), ice chips or chew gum if your mouth becomes dry. It is especially important to brush your teeth regularly if you develop a dry mouth.

Do not stop taking this medicine suddenly without the approval of your doctor.

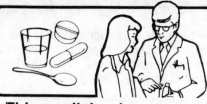

Conjugated Estrogens

Common Trade Names:
Premarin

This medicine has many uses and the reason it was prescribed depends on your condition. If you do not understand why you are taking it, check with your doctor.

The tablets may be taken after meals or with a snack if they upset your stomach.

Vaginal cream:
1. Remove cap from tube of medication.
2. Screw applicator to tube.
3. Gently squeeze the tube of cream to force the prescribed amount into the applicator.
4. Unscrew the applicator from the tube of medication.

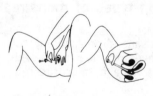

5. Hold the applicator by the cylinder and gently insert into the vaginal canal as far as it will comfortably go.
6. While still holding the cylinder, press plunger gently to deposit medication.
7. While keeping plunger depressed, remove applicator from vaginal canal.

8. After each use, take the applicator apart and wash thoroughly with warm water and soap and rinse thoroughly. Allow to dry.

9. Reassemble the applicator.

Contact your doctor if you develop any of the following:
Severe or persistent headache.
Blurred vision, dizziness or faintness.
Pain in calves of legs.
Weight gain or swelling of hands or ankles.

Chest pain or shortness of breath or coughing of blood. In women, irregular or missed menstrual period, unusual vaginal bleeding or lumps in the breast.
Skin rash or yellowing of the skin or eyes.

If you are pregnant or think you may be pregnant, contact your doctor.

A more detailed leaflet is available with your prescription. If you have any questions or need help to understand the leaflet, ask your doctor or pharmacist.

Combination Estrogen-Progestogen Therapy (21 day)

Common Trade Names: Demulen, Lo/Ovral, Norinyl 1/50 21, Norlestrin-21, Ortho Novum 1/80 21, Ortho Novum 1/50 21, Ovral, Ovulen-21

This medicine is used as a birth control measure and to treat hormonal disorders. Some products are also used to treat certain types of menstrual problems.

Take this drug at the same time each day, for example, after the evening meal or at bedtime. It is important to take this drug regularly.

Consult your doctor if any of the following side effects occur:
1. Severe or persistent headache.
2. Vomiting, dizziness, fainting.
3. Blurred vision or slurred speech.

4. Pain in the calves of the legs or numbness in an arm or leg.
5. Chest pain, shortness of breath or coughing of blood.
6. Lumps in the breast.
7. Severe depression.
8. Yellowing of the skin.
9. Severe abdominal pain.
10. Breakthrough bleeding which persists

after the third month of therapy. During the first 3 months of therapy, breakthrough bleeding may be expected, but you should keep taking the tablets and it will usually clear up in a day or two.

11. If you miss two consecutive menstrual periods or if you think you are pregnant.

It is recommended that you do not smoke while you are on this drug.

Contact your doctor at least once every 6-12 months so that he can examine you.

If you are taking this drug for birth control, take the tablets as follows:

1. During the first month of taking this drug it is important to use some additional form of birth control to help prevent pregnancy.

2. The first day of menstruation is day **one.** Begin taking this medication on day **five** of your menstrual cycle. Write this day in the space provided on the package. The day of the week that you take your first tablet is your regular starting day for future cycles.

3. Take one tablet every day for three weeks (21 days). Take it at the same time every day — preferably after dinner or at bedtime.

4. After finishing the package of 21 tablets, wait 7 days. Do not take any tablets during these days. Your period will probably start about three days after you took the last tablet.

5. On the 8th day, start a new package of 21 tablets and again take one tablet daily. It is important to start taking your tablets on your original starting day whether or not menstruation occurs as expected.

6. Repeat this 21 days on and 7 days off cycle.

If Menstruation Starts On	Start Tablets On
Sunday	Thursday
Monday	Friday
Tuesday	Saturday
Wednesday	Sunday
Thursday	Monday
Friday	Tuesday
Saturday	Wednesday

Day 5 of first cycle Take 1st Tablet

7. If you miss one daily dose, take it as soon as you remember and continue your regular schedule. If you miss two daily doses, take 2 tablets daily for the next 2 days then resume your normal schedule. It is advisable to use some additional form of birth control for at least the next seven days to help avoid pregnancy.

8. If you miss 3 daily doses, stop taking the medication and discard the remainder of the package. Start a new schedule of tablets on the 8th day after the last dose was taken. An additional form of birth control should be used until the start of the next menstrual period. Call the doctor if there is any chance that you may be pregnant.

9. Call your doctor if you do not have a period within 45 days of your last menstrual period to rule out the chance that you may be pregnant.

A more detailed leaflet is available with your prescription. If you have any questions or need help to understand the leaflet, ask your doctor or pharmacist.

Combination Estrogen-Progestogen Therapy (28 day)
Common Trade Names:
Ovral-28

This medicine is used as a birth control measure and to treat hormonal disorders.

Take this drug at the same time each day, for example, after the evening meal or at bedtime. It is important to take this drug regularly.

Consult your doctor if any of the following side effects occur:
1. Severe or persistent headache.
2. Vomiting, dizziness, fainting.
3. Blurred vision or slurred speech.

4. Pain in the calves of the legs or numbness in an arm or leg.

5. Chest pain, shortness of breath or coughing of blood.

6. Lumps in the breast.

7. Severe depression.

8. Yellowing of the skin.

9. Severe abdominal pain.

10. Breakthrough bleeding which persists after the third month of therapy. During the first 3 months of therapy, breakthrough bleeding may be expected, but you should keep taking the tablets and it will usually clear up in a day or two.

11. If you miss two consecutive menstrual periods or if you think you are pregnant.

It is recommended that you do not smoke while you are on this drug.

Contact your doctor at least once every 6-12 months so that he can examine you.

If you are taking this drug for birth control, take the tablets as follows:

2. The first day of menstruation is day **one.** Begin taking this medication on day **five** of your menstrual cycle.

3. Take one tablet every day for 28 days. Take it at the same time every day — perferably after dinner or at bedtime. Take the tablets in numerical sequence. Do not miss a day between tablets. The first 21 tablets you take will contain active ingredients and the last 7 tablets contain no active ingredients. They are simply included to make it more convenient for you. You will probably have your period while you are taking these last 7 tablets.

4. After finishing the package, start a new package of 28 tablets the next day. Do not miss a day between finishing one package and starting another. It is important to take this medication regularly whether or not menstruation occurs as expected.

If Menstruation Starts On	Start Tablets On
Sunday	Thursday
Monday	Friday

Tuesday . . . . Saturday
Wednesday . . . . Sunday
Thursday . . . . Monday
Friday . . . . Tuesday
Saturday . . . . Wednesday

5. If you miss one daily dose, take it as soon as you remember and continue your regular schedule. If you miss two daily doses take 2 tablets daily for the next 2 days then resume your normal schedule. It is advisable to use some additional form of birth control for at least the next seven days to help avoid pregnancy.

6. If you miss 3 daily doses, stop taking the medication and discard the remainder of the package. Start a new schedule of tablets on the 8th day after the last dose was taken. An additional form of birth control should be used until the start of the next menstrual period. Call your doctor if there is any chance that you may be pregnant.

7. Call your doctor if you do not have a period within 45 days of your last menstrual period to rule out the chance that you may be pregnant.

A more detailed leaflet is available with your prescription. If you have any questions or need help to understand the leaflet, ask your doctor or pharmacist.

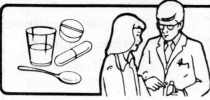

Cyproheptadine

Common Trade Names:
Periactin

 This medicine is used to help relieve symptoms (such as itching) of certain types of allergic conditions.

 This drug may be taken with food if it upsets your stomach.

 In some people, this drug may cause dizziness or drowsiness. Do not drive a car or operate dangerous machinery or do jobs that require you to be alert until you know how you are going to react to this drug.

 If you become dizzy, you should be careful going up and down stairs. Sit or lie down at the first sign of dizziness.

 Do not drink alcoholic beverages while taking this drug.

 It is important that you obtain the advice of your doctor before taking pain relievers, non-prescription drugs, sleeping pills or tranquilizers while you are taking this drug.

 Suck a hard sour candy (sugarless), ice chips or chew gum if your mouth becomes dry. It is especially important to brush your teeth regularly if you develop a dry mouth.

 Call your doctor if you develop a sore throat, fever, mouth sores or a skin rash.

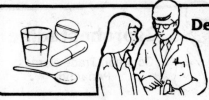

Dexbrompheniramine-
Pseudoephedrine

Common Trade Names:
Drixoral

This medicine is used to help relieve the symptoms of nasal stuffiness and certain types of allergic conditions.

This drug may be taken with food if it upsets your stomach.

Swallow the tablets whole. Do not crush, chew or break them into pieces.

In some people, this drug may cause dizziness or drowsiness. Do not drive a car or operate dangerous machinery or do jobs that require you to be alert until you know how you are going to react to this drug.

If you become dizzy, you should be careful going up and down stairs. Sit or lie down at the first sign of dizziness.

Do not drink alcoholic beverages while taking this drug.

It is important that you obtain the advice of your doctor before taking pain relievers, non-prescription drugs, sleeping pills or tranquilizers while you are taking this drug.

Call your doctor if you develop blurred vision, weakness, fast heart rate, insomnia or unusual nervousness.

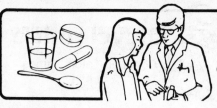

Diazepam

Common Trade Names:
Valium

This medicine is used to help relieve anxiety and tension. It is also used to help relax muscles and to treat some conditions of the nerves.

In some people, this drug may cause dizziness or drowsiness. Do not drive a car or operate dangerous machinery or do jobs that require you to be alert until you know how you are going to react to this drug.

If you become dizzy, you should be careful going up and down stairs. Sit or lie down at the first sign of dizziness.

Do not drink alcoholic beverages while taking this drug or for a few days after you have stopped taking the drug.

It is important that you obtain the advice of your doctor before taking pain relievers, non-prescription drugs, sleeping pills or tranquilizers while you are taking this drug.

Do not take any more of this drug than your doctor has prescribed and do not stop taking this medicine without the approval of your doctor.

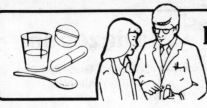

Dicyclomine

Common Trade Names
Bentyl

This medicine is used to help relax muscles in the stomach and intestines.

Take the medicine 30 minutes before a meal unless otherwise directed.

If the SYRUP form of the drug has been prescribed for a baby, the syrup may be diluted with an equal amount of water.

In some people, this drug may cause drowsiness or blurred vision. Do not drive a car or operate dangerous machinery or do jobs that require you to be alert until you know how you are going to react to this drug.

Suck a hard sour candy (sugarless), ice chips or chew gum if your mouth becomes dry. It is especially important to brush your teeth regularly if you develop a dry mouth.

Try to avoid exercise or hard work in very warm temperatures as this drug makes some people more sensitive to heat and may cause fainting.

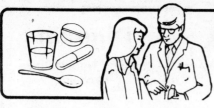

Diethylpropion

Common Trade Names:
Tenuate, Tepanil

 This medicine is used to decrease the appetite in weight reduction programs.

It is important that you follow the diet prescribed by your doctor.

 If you were prescribed TENUATE DOSPAN or TEPANIL TENTAB, swallow the tablets whole. Do not crush, chew or break them into pieces.

Do not take any more of this drug than your doctor has prescribed and do not stop taking it suddenly without first asking your doctor.

 In some people, this drug may cause dizziness or drowsiness. Do not drive a car or operate dangerous machinery or do jobs that require you to be alert until you know how you are going to react to this drug.

 If you become dizzy, you should be careful going up and down stairs. Sit or lie down at the first sign of dizziness.

 Suck a hard sour candy (sugarless), ice chips or chew gum if your mouth becomes dry. It is especially important to brush your teeth regularly if you develop a dry mouth.

 Call your doctor if you develop a sore throat, fever, mouth sores, skin rash or fast heart rate.

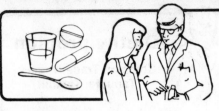

Digoxin

Common Trade Names:
Lanoxin

This medicine is used to help make the heart beat strong and steady.

It is very important that you take this drug as your doctor has prescribed and that you do not miss any doses. Take this medicine at the same time every day and do not go without this medicine between prescription refills.

If a dropper is used to measure the liquid dose and you do not fully understand how to use it, check with your pharmacist.

Some non-prescription drugs, especially cough and cold remedies, may aggravate your condition. Read the label of the product you select to see if there is a warning. If there is, check with your doctor or pharmacist before using it.

Call your doctor immediately if you develop a slow or irregular pulse, nausea, vomiting, diarrhea (loose bowel movements), loss of appetite, unusual weakness, blurred vision or changes in color vision.

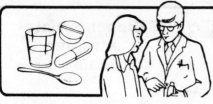

Diphenhydramine

Common Trade Names:
**Benadryl, Benadryl Elixir,
Benylin Cough Syrup**

This medicine has many uses and the reason it was prescribed depends on your condition. If you do not fully understand why you are taking it, check with your doctor.

This medicine may be taken with food if it upsets your stomach.

Suck a hard sour candy (sugarless), ice chips or chew gum if your mouth becomes dry. It is especially important to brush your teeth regularly if you develop a dry mouth.

In some people, this drug may cause dizziness or drowsiness. Do not drive a car or operate dangerous machinery or do jobs that require you to be alert until you know how you are going to react to this drug. If you become dizzy, you should be careful going up and down stairs. Sit or lie down at the first sign of dizziness.

Do not drink alcoholic beverages while taking this drug.

It is important that you obtain the advice of your doctor before taking pain relievers, nonprescription drugs, sleeping pills or tranquilizers while you are taking this drug.

Do not use this medicine more often or longer than recommended by your doctor.

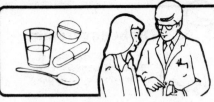

Diphenoxylate-Atropine

Common Trade Names:
Lomotil

This medicine is used to treat diarrhea (loose bowel movements).

Do not use this medicine more often or longer than prescribed by your doctor. The body has warning signs if you take too much of this medicine. Call your doctor if you develop a fever, fast heart beat, difficulty in breathing, rapid eye movements or convulsions.

For Liquid Medicine:

Use the special dropper that comes with the medicine. If you have any questions about how to use it, ask your pharmacist.

Drink plenty of water each day to help replace the fluids which have been lost due to diarrhea unless otherwise directed by your doctor.

In some people this drug may cause dizziness or drowsiness. Do not drive a car or operate dangerous machinery or do jobs that require you to be alert until you know how you are going to react to this drug. If you become dizzy, you should be careful going up and down stairs. Sit or lie down at the first sign of dizziness.

Do not drink alcoholic beverages while taking this drug.

It is important that you obtain the advice of your doctor before taking pain relievers, non-prescription drugs, sleeping pills or tranquilizers while you are taking this drug.

Call your doctor if you develop bloating or vomiting or if the diarrhea continues.

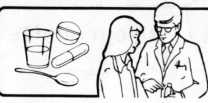

Dipyridamole

Common Trade Names
Persantine

This medicine is usually used to help prevent or relieve chest pain.

Take this medicine on an empty stomach at least 1 hour before meals with a full 8-ounce glass of milk or water. The drug may be taken with a light snack if it upsets your stomach.

In some people, this drug may cause flushing of the face or dizziness. Sit or lie down until these effects pass. Do not drive a car or operate dangerous machinery or do jobs that require you to be alert if you are dizzy.

You may have to take this medicine for 2 or 3 months before you feel its full benefit.

Some non-prescription drugs, especially cough and cold remedies, may aggravate your condition. Read the label of the product you select to see if there is a warning. If there is, check with your doctor or pharmacist before using it.

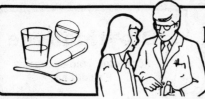

Disopyramide

Common Trade Names
Norpace

This medicine is used to make the heart beat at a normal rate.

It is very important that you take this medicine as your doctor has directed and that you do not miss any doses. Take this medicine at the same times every day and do not go without this drug between prescription refills.

In some people, this drug may cause dizziness or blurred vision. Do not drive a car or operate dangerous machinery or do jobs that require you to be alert until you know how you are going to react to the drug.

If you become dizzy, you should be careful going up and down stairs and you should not change positions too rapidly. Get out of bed slowly in the morning and dangle your feet over the edge of the bed for a few minutes before standing up. Sit or lie down at the first sign of dizziness. Tell your doctor you have been dizzy.

Suck a hard sour candy (sugarless), ice chips or chew gum if your mouth becomes dry. It is especially important to brush your teeth regularly if you develop a dry mouth.

Some non-prescription drugs, especially cough and cold remedies, may aggravate your condition. Read the label of the product you select to see if there is a warning. If there is, check with your doctor or pharmacist before using it.

Call your doctor if you have difficulty urinating ("passing your water") or if you develop shortness of breath or chest pain.

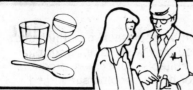

Doxepin

Common Trade Names:
Sinequan

This medicine is used to help relieve the symptoms of depression and anxiety.

The full effect of this medicine will not be noticed immediately but may take from a few days to four weeks.

In some people, this drug may cause dizziness or drowsiness. Do not drive a car or operate dangerous machinery or do jobs that require you to be alert until you know how you are going to react to this drug.

If this medicine causes dizziness, you should be careful going up and down stairs and you should not change positions too rapidly. Get out of bed slowly in the morning and dangle your feet over the edge of the bed for a few minutes before standing. Sit or lie down at the first sign of dizziness. Tell your doctor you have been dizzy.

Do not drink alcoholic beverages while taking this drug.

It is important that you obtain the advice of your doctor before taking pain relievers, non-prescription drugs, sleeping pills or tranquilizers while you are taking this drug.

Suck a hard sour candy (sugarless), ice chips or chew gum if your mouth becomes dry. It is especially important to brush your teeth regularly if you develop a dry mouth.

This medicine makes some people more sensitive to sunlight or sunlamps. If your skin becomes more sensitive to sunlight, tell your doctor and try to stay out of direct sunlight.

While in the sun, wear protective clothing and sunglasses. You may wish to ask your pharmacist about suitable sunscreen products. Call your doctor if you become sunburned.

Do not stop taking this medicine suddenly without the approval of your doctor.

Call your doctor if you develop a sore throat, fever, mouth sores, eye pain, or difficulty in urinating (passing your water).

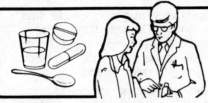

Doxycycline

Vibramycin

Minocycline

Minocin, Vectrin

This medicine is an antibiotic used to treat certain types of infections and skin conditions.

If you develop stomach upset after taking the drug, take it with a snack. Call your doctor if you continue to have stomach upset.

For Liquid Medicines:

Shake the bottle well each time you use it so that you can measure an accurate dose.

If there is a discard date on the bottle, throw away any unused medicine after that date. Do not take or save old medicine. Call your pharmacist if you are not sure of the discard date.

It is important to take **all** of this medicine plus any refills that your doctor told you to take. Do not stop taking it earlier than your doctor has recommended in spite of the fact that you may feel better. Otherwise, the infection may return.

If you must take iron products or vitamins containing iron, take them 2 hours before (or 3 hours after) this medicine.

Some antacids can make this medicine less effective if they are taken at the same time. If you must take antacids, they should be taken at least 3 hours after this medicine. If you have any questions, ask your pharmacist.

This medicine makes some people more sensitive to sunlight or sunlamps. If your skin becomes more sensitive to sunlight, tell your doctor and try to stay out of direct sunlight. While in the sun, wear protective clothing and sunglasses. You may wish to ask your pharmacist about suitable sunscreen products. Call your doctor if you become sunburned.

Call your doctor if you develop a skin rash, sore mouth, troublesome diarrhea (loose bowel movements), or (in women) a vaginal discharge which was not present before you started taking this medicine.

If for some reason you cannot take all of the medicine, discard the unused portion by flushing it down the toilet. Do not save this medicine for future use because outdated tetracycline can cause serious problems.

In some people, MINOCYCLINE may cause dizziness. Do not drive a car or operate dangerous machinery or do jobs that require you to be alert until you know how you are going to react to this drug. Call your doctor if the dizziness does not disappear.

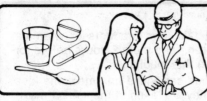

Doxylamine-Pyridoxine
Common Trade Names:
Bendectin

 This medicine is used to treat the nausea and vomiting of pregnancy.

 In some people, this drug may cause dizziness or drowsiness. Do not drive a car or operate dangerous machinery or do jobs that require you to be alert until you know how you are going to react to this drug.

 If you become dizzy, you should be careful going up and down stairs. Sit or lie down at the first sign of dizziness.

 Do not drink alcoholic beverages while taking this drug.

 It is important that you obtain the advice of your doctor before taking pain relievers, nonprescription drugs, sleeping pills or tranquilizers while you are taking this drug.

This medicine must be swallowed whole. Do not crush, chew or break it into pieces.

 Call your doctor if you develop nervousness, headache, fast heart rate or troublesome diarrhea.

Erythromycin
E-Mycin, Erythromycin Base
Erythromycin Estolate
Ilosone

Erythromycin Ethyl Succinate
E.E.S., Pediamycin
Erythromycin Stearate
Erythrocin Stearate

This medicine is an antibiotic used to treat certain types of infections.

The way you take your medicine will depend on the type of drug your doctor prescribed. If you received:

Erythromycin Base Tablets, Erythrocin Filmtabs

• It is best to take this medicine with a glass of water on an empty stomach at least 1 hour before (or 2 hours after) eating food. Take it at the proper time even if you skip a meal. If you develop stomach upset after taking the drug, take it with some food. Call your doctor if you continue to have an upset stomach.

E.E.S., Ilosone, Pediamycin

• The medicine may be taken with a glass of water on an empty stomach or with food.

E-Mycin

• These tablets have a special coating and must be swallowed whole. Do not crush, chew or break them into pieces. Take with a glass of water on an empty stomach or with food.

Erythrocin Chewable Tablets, Ilosone Chewable Tablets, Pediamycin Chewable Tablets

• Chew the tablets well before swallowing. Do not swallow the tablets whole.

For Liquid Medicines:
• Store the bottle of medicine in a refrigerator but do not freeze.

● Each time you use it, shake the bottle well so that you can measure an accurate dose.

● If a dropper is used to measure the dose and you do not fully understand how to use it, check with your pharmacist.

● If there is a discard date on the bottle, throw away any unused medicine after that date. Do not take or save old medicine. Call your pharmacist if you are not sure of the discard date.

It is important to take **all** of this medicine plus any refills that your doctor told you to take. Do not stop taking this medicine earlier than your doctor has recommended in spite of the fact that you feel better. Otherwise, the infection may return.

This medicine sometimes causes diarrhea (loose bowel movements). Call your doctor if the diarrhea becomes severe or does not go away after a few days.

If you are taking ILOSONE and develop severe stomach cramps, nausea, vomiting, fever or yellow color of the skin or eyes, call your doctor.

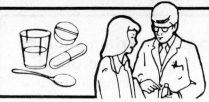

Fenoprofen

Common Trade Names:
Nalfon

This medicine is used to help relieve pain, redness and swelling in certain kinds of arthritis and other medical conditions.

The full effect of this medicine will not be noticed immediately but may take from a few days to 3 weeks.

It is best to take this medicine on an empty stomach at least 1 hour before (or 2 hours after) food unless otherwise directed. If you develop stomach upset, take the drug with food or immediately after meals or with an antacid. Call your doctor if you continue to have stomach upset.

In some people, this drug may cause dizziness or drowsiness. Do not drive a car or operate dangerous machinery or do jobs that require you to be alert until you know how you are going to react to this drug.

If you become dizzy, you should be careful going up and down stairs. Sit or lie down at the first sign of dizziness.

Call your doctor if you develop a skin rash, "ringing" or "buzzing" in the ears, fast heart beats, swelling of the ankles, blurred vision, black stools or severe stomach pain.

Fluocinonide Triamcinolone
Lidex
Acetonide
Aristocort, Kenalog

This drug is used to help relieve pain, itching, redness and swelling of certain types of skin conditions.

Instructions For Use:

1. Cleanse the skin area well with soap and water unless otherwise directed by your doctor. Allow the skin to dry completely or pat dry with a clean towel.

2. Apply the drug to the affected area and rub in lightly. Do not bandage unless directed by your doctor.

Do not use the drug more frequently or in larger quantities than prescribed by your doctor.

Do not apply cosmetics or lotions on top of the drug unless your doctor approves.

Call your doctor if the condition for which this medication is being used persists or becomes worse, or if it causes a constant irritation such as itching or burning.

For external use only. Keep this drug away from the eyes.

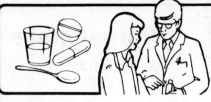

Flurazepam

Common Trade Names:
Dalmane

This medicine is a sleeping pill.

If this medicine causes drowsiness or dizziness the next day after you take it, do not drive a car or operate dangerous machinery or do jobs that require you to be alert. If this "hangover" drowsiness becomes bothersome, call your doctor.

If you are dizzy the next day, you should be careful going up and down stairs. Sit or lie down at the first sign of dizziness.

Do not drink alcoholic beverages while taking this drug.

It is important that you obtain the advice of your doctor before taking pain relievers, non-prescription drugs, other sleeping pills or tranquilizers while you are taking this drug.

Do not take any more of this drug than your doctor has prescribed and go to bed after you have taken it.

Do not smoke in bed after taking this sleeping pill.

Call your doctor if you develop bothersome nightmares or sleepiness during the day.

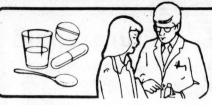

Furosemide

Common Trade Names:
Lasix

This medicine is used to help rid the body of excess fluids, decrease swelling and to treat high blood pressure. It is commonly called a "water pill".

It is very important that you take the medicine as your doctor has directed. Try to remember to take all your doses.

Take this medicine at the same time each day. When you first start taking this medicine, you will probably urinate (pass your water) more often and in larger amounts than usual. Therefore, do not initially take it at bedtime or you may have to get up during the night to go to the bathroom.

This drug may be taken with food or milk if it upsets your stomach.

This medicine normally causes your body to lose potassium. The body has warning signs to let you know if too much potassium is being lost. Call your doctor if you become unusually thirsty or if you develop leg cramps or unusual weakness, dizziness, fatigue, vomiting or confusion. Your doctor may prescribe some medicine to replace the potassium or he may tell you to eat foods which contain a lot of potassium (for example, orange juice, bananas, dates, raisins).

If this medicine causes dizziness, you should be careful going up and down stairs and you should not change positions too rapidly. Get out of bed slowly in the morning and dangle your feet over the edge of the bed for a few minutes before standing up. Sit down or lie down at the first sign of dizziness. Call your doctor and tell him you have been dizzy. Be careful drinking alcoholic beverages while taking this medicine because it can make this dizziness worse. Do not drive a car or operate dangerous machinery if you are dizzy.

Call your doctor if you develop a sore throat, fever, or sharp joint pain.

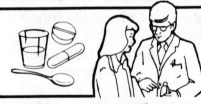

Hydralazine

Common Trade Names:
Apresoline

This medicine is used to lower blood pressure.

It is very important that you take this medicine as your doctor has directed and that you do not miss any doses. Hypertension (high blood pressure) is a longterm disease and it may be necessary for you to take the drug for a long time in spite of the fact that you feel better. Do not go without medicine between prescription refills.

Take the medicine with food or milk.

Headaches may occur during the first few days and then will usually disappear within the first week. If they continue, call your doctor.

63

If this medicine causes dizziness, you should be careful going up and down stairs and you should not change positions too rapidly. Get out of bed slowly in the morning and dangle your feet over the edge of the bed for a few minutes before standing up. Sit or lie down at the first sign of dizziness. Tell your doctor you have been dizzy.

Call your doctor if you develop a sore throat, fever, mouth sores, fast heart beat, sharp joint pain or a skin rash.

Hydrochlorothiazide
Esidrix, HydroDIURIL
Chlorthalidone
Hygroton

Chlorothiazide
Diuril
Methychlothiazide
Enduron

This medicine is used to help rid the body of excess fluids, decrease swelling and to treat high blood pressure. It is commonly called a "water pill".

It is very important that you take the medicine as your doctor has directed. Try to remember to take all your doses.

Take this medicine at the same time each day. When you first start taking this medicine, you will probably urinate (pass your water) more often and in larger amounts than usual. Therefore, do not initially take it at bedtime or you may have to get up during the night to go to the bathroom.

This drug may be taken with food or milk if it upsets your stomach.

This medicine normally causes your body to lose potassium. The body has warning signs to let you know if too much potassium is being lost. Call your doctor if you become unusually thirsty or if you develop leg cramps or unusual weakness, dizziness, fatigue, vomiting or confusion. Your doctor may prescribe some medicine to replace the potassium or he may tell you to eat foods which contain a lot of potassium (for example, orange juice, bananas, dates, raisins).

If this medicine causes dizziness, you should be careful going up and down stairs and you should not change positions too rapidly. Get out of bed slowly in the morning and dangle your feet over the edge of the bed for a few minutes before standing up. Sit down or lie down at the first sign of dizziness. Call your doctor and tell him you have been dizzy. Be careful drinking alcoholic beverages while taking this medicine because it can make this dizziness worse. Do not drive a car or operate dangerous machinery if you are dizzy.

This medicine may make some people more sensitive to sunlight and sunlamps. If your skin becomes more sensitive to sunlight, tell your doctor and try to stay out of direct sunlight. While in the sun, wear protective clothing and sunglasses. You may wish to ask your pharmacist about suitable sunscreen products. Call your doctor if you become sunburned.

Call your doctor if you develop sharp joint pain, sore throat or fever.

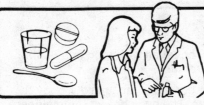

Hydroxyzine

Common Trade Names:
Atarax, Vistaril

 This medicine is used to help relieve the symptoms of anxiety and tension and certain types of emotional problems. This drug has several other uses and the reason it was prescribed depends upon your condition. Check with your doctor if you do not fully understand why you are taking it.

 In some people, this drug may cause drowsiness. Do not drive a car or operate dangerous machinery or do jobs that require you to be alert until you know how you are going to react to this drug.

 Do not drink alcoholic beverages while taking this drug.

 It is important that you obtain the advice of your doctor before taking pain relievers, non-prescription drugs, sleeping pills or tranquilizers while you are taking this drug.

 Suck a hard sour candy (sugarless), ice chips or chew gum if your mouth becomes dry. It is especially important to brush your teeth regularly if you develop a dry mouth.

 Call your doctor if you develop a sore throat, fever, mouth sores or skin rash.

66

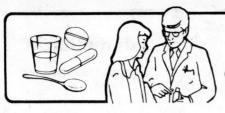

Ibuprofen

Common Trade Names:
Motrin

This medicine is used to help relieve pain. It is also used to help relieve redness and swelling in certain kinds of arthritis.

It is best to take this medicine on an empty stomach. If you develop stomach upset after taking the drug, take it with some food.

You may have to take this medicine for 1-2 weeks before you feel its full benefits.

In some people this drug may cause dizziness. Do not drive a car or operate dangerous machinery or do jobs that require you to be alert until you know how you are going to react to this drug.

If you become dizzy, you should be careful going up and down stairs. Sit or lie down at the first sign of dizziness.

Call your doctor if you develop "ringing" or "buzzing" in the ears, skin rash, stomach pain, black stools, blurred vision, weight gain or swelling of the ankles.

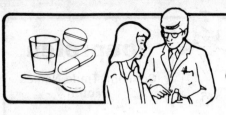

Indomethacin

Common Trade Names:
Indocin

This medicine is used to help relieve pain, redness and swelling in certain kinds of arthritis and other medical conditions.

Always take the drug with food or immediately after meals or with an antacid.

It is important to take this medicine regularly and continuously since it may take several weeks before its benefits are noticed.

This medicine may cause headaches which will usually disappear with continued use. Call your doctor if they continue.

In some people this drug may cause dizziness or drowsiness. Do not drive a car or operate dangerous machinery or do jobs that require you to be alert until you know how you are going to react to this drug. If you become dizzy, you should be careful going up and down stairs. Sit or lie down at the first sign of dizziness.

Contact your doctor if you develop a skin rash, sore throat, fever, mouth sores, black stools, diarrhea (loose bowel movements), stomach pain, blurred vision or depression.

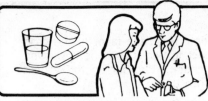

Isosorbide

Common Trade Names:
Isordil, Sorbitrate

This medicine is used to help relieve or prevent a type of chest pain called angina.

The way you take your medicine will depend on the type of drug your doctor prescribed. If you received:

Oral Tablets

This medicine should be swallowed. Take on an empty stomach unless otherwise directed.

Sublingual Tablets

This medicine should NOT be swallowed. This medicine should be used at the first sign of an attack of angina.

Place tablet under the tongue until it is completely dissolved.

Do not swallow until the drug has dissolved and do not rinse the mouth for a few minutes. Do not take additional doses unless your doctor has directed.

If your chest pain is not relieved within 15 minutes, call your doctor immediately.

Chewable Tablets

Chew the tablets well before swallowing. Take on an empty stomach unless otherwise directed.

Sustained Action Tablets and Capsules

Swallow this medicine whole. Do not chew or crush. Take on an empty stomach unless otherwise directed.

Some non-prescription drugs, especially cough and cold remedies, may aggravate your condition. Read the label of the product you select to see if there is a warning. If there is, check with your doctor or pharmacist before using it.

During the first few days of using this medicine you may experience a headache. It may be relieved by taking the drug with some food or if your doctor agrees, by taking aspirin. This is a normal side effect and it usually disappears within a few days. Call your doctor if it continues.

If this medicine causes dizziness, you should be careful going up and down stairs, and you should not change positions too rapidly. Get out of bed slowly in the morning and dangle your feet over the edge of the bed for a few minutes before standing up. Sit or lie down at the first sign of dizziness. Do not drive a car or operate machinery.

Do not drink alcoholic beverages while taking this drug because the combination may cause undesired side effects.

It is recommended that you carry an identification card indicating that you are taking this medicine.

Contact your doctor if you develop a skin rash.

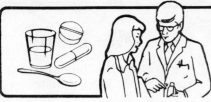

Isoxsuprine

Common Trade Names:
Vasodilan

This medicine is used in certain types of conditions to help improve the flow of blood to cells of the body.

In some people, this drug may cause dizziness. Do not drive a car or operate dangerous machinery or do jobs that require you to be alert until you know how you are going to react to this drug.

If this medicine causes dizziness, you should be careful going up and down stairs and you should not change positions too rapidly. Get out of bed slowly in the morning and dangle your feet over the edge of the bed for a few minutes before standing up. Sit or lie down at the first sign of dizziness. Tell your doctor you have been dizzy.

Call your doctor if you develop a skin rash or fast heart rate.

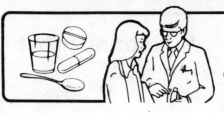

Meclizine

Common Trade Names:
Antivert, Bonine

 This medicine is used to treat nausea, vomiting and dizziness and to help prevent motion sickness.

 If you were prescribed CHEWABLE TABLETS, you should chew them well before swallowing. Do not swallow them whole.

 Suck a hard sour candy (sugarless), ice chips or chew gum if your mouth becomes dry. It is especially important to brush your teeth regularly if you develop a dry mouth.

 In some people, this drug may cause drowsiness or blurred vision. Do not drive a car or operate dangerous machinery or do jobs that require you to be alert until you know how you are going to react to this medicine.

 Do not drink alcoholic beverages while taking this drug.

 It is important that you obtain the advice of your doctor before taking pain relievers, non-prescription drugs, sleeping pills or tranquilizers while you are taking this drug.

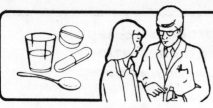

Meprobamate

Common Trade Names:
**Equanil, Meprospan,
Miltown, SK-Bamate**

This medicine is used to help relieve anxiety and tension.

If you were prescribed MEPROSPAN, swallow the capsules whole. Do not crush, chew or mash the contents.

In some people, this drug may cause dizziness or drowsiness. Do not drive a car or operate dangerous machinery or do jobs that require you to be alert until you know how you are going to react to this drug.

If you become dizzy, you should be careful going up and down stairs. Sit or lie down at the first sign of dizziness.

Do not drink alcoholic beverages while taking this drug.

It is important that you obtain the advice of your doctor before taking pain relievers, nonprescription drugs, sleeping pills or tranquilizers while you are taking this drug.

Do not stop taking this medicine suddenly without the approval of your doctor.

Call your doctor if you develop a sore throat, fever, mouth sores or skin rash.

Meprobamate-Aspirin-Ethoheptazine

Common Trade Names:
Equagesic

This medicine is used to help relieve pain and tension.

Do not take this medicine more often or longer than your doctor has prescribed.

In some people, this drug may cause dizziness or drowsiness. Do not drive a car or operate dangerous machinery or do jobs that require you to be alert until you know how you are going to react to this drug.

If you become dizzy, you should be careful going up and down stairs. Sit or lie down at the first sign of dizziness.

Do not drink alcoholic beverages while taking this drug.

It is important that you obtain the advice of your doctor before taking other pain relievers, non-prescription drugs, sleeping pills or tranquilizers while you are taking this drug.

Do not stop taking this medicine suddenly without the approval of your doctor.

Call your doctor if you develop a sore throat, fever, mouth sores, skin rash.

Do not take or save old medicine. Throw away this medicine if it smells like vinegar.

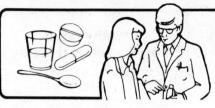

Methyldopa

Common Trade Names:
Aldomet

This medicine is used to lower the blood pressure.

It is very important that you take this medicine as your doctor has directed and that you do not miss any doses. Hypertension (high blood pressure) is a longterm disease and it may be necessary for you to take the drug for a long time in spite of the fact that you feel better. Do not go without medicine between prescription refills.

Drowsiness may occur during the first 2 or 3 days and then will usually disappear. Do not drive a car or operate dangerous machinery or do jobs that require you to be alert until you know how you are going to react to this drug. Be careful drinking alcoholic beverages because they could make the drowsiness worse.

If this medicine causes dizziness, you should be careful going up and down stairs and you should not change positions too rapidly. Get out of bed slowly in the morning and dangle your feet over the edge of the bed for a few minutes before standing up. Sit or lie down at the first sign of dizziness. Tell your doctor you have been dizzy.

Call your doctor if you develop a sore throat, fever, or skin rash.

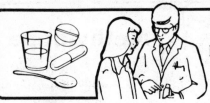

Methyldopa-Hydrochlorothiazide

Common Trade Names:
Aldoril

This medicine is used to lower the blood pressure.

It is very important that you take this medicine as your doctor has directed and that you do not miss any doses. Hypertension (high blood pressure) is a longterm disease and it may be necessary for you to take the drug for a long time in spite of the fact that you feel better. Do not go without medicine between prescription refills.

This medicine normally causes your body to lose potassium. The body has warning signs to let you know if too much potassium is being lost. Call your doctor if you become unusually thirsty or if you develop leg cramps or unusual weakness, fatigue, vomiting or confusion. Your doctor may prescribe some medicine to replace the potassium or he may tell you to eat foods which contain a lot of potassium (for example, orange juice, bananas, dates, raisins).

This medicine may make some people more sensitive to sunlight and sunlamps. If your skin becomes more sensitive to sunlight, tell your doctor and try to stay out of direct sunlight. While in the sun, wear protective clothing and sunglasses. You may wish to ask your pharmacist about suitable sunscreen products. Call your doctor if you become sunburned.

Drowsiness may occur during the first 2 or 3 days and then will usually disappear. Do not drive a car or operate dangerous machinery or do jobs that require you to be alert until you know how you are going to react to this drug. Be careful drinking alcoholic beverages because they could make the drowsiness worse.

If this medicine causes dizziness, you should be careful going up and down stairs and you should not change positions too rapidly. Get out of bed slowly in the morning and dangle your feet over the edge of the bed for a few minutes before standing up. Sit or lie down at the first sign of dizziness. Tell your doctor you have been dizzy.

Call your doctor if you develop sharp joint pain, sore throat, fever, or a skin rash.

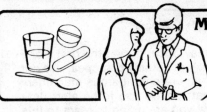

Methylprednisolone
Medrol Oral
Prednisone
Deltasone, Meticorten, Paracort

This medicine is similar to a hormone called cortisone that is produced by the body. This medicine has many uses and the reason it was prescribed depends upon your condition. If you do not understand why you are taking it, check with your doctor.

Take the drug after meals or with a snack if it upsets your stomach. Call your doctor if you continue to have an upset stomach (especially if it awakens you during the night) or if your stools become black and tarry.

It is very important that you take this drug as your doctor has prescribed. Take it at the same time every day and do not go without medicine between prescription refills.

Do not stop taking this medicine suddenly without the approval of your doctor.

Bruising may occur more easily. Try to protect yourself from all injuries to prevent bruising.

Call your doctor if you develop nightmares or a change in your mood, sore throat, fever, swelling of legs and ankles, an infection that does not clear up as quickly as usual, dizziness, weakness or muscle pain or changes in vision.

Tell every doctor and dentist who treats you that you are taking this medicine.

Carry a card in your wallet or wear a bracelet stating that you are taking this drug.

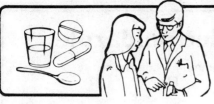

Metoprolol

Common Trade Names
Lopressor

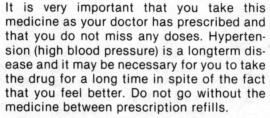

This medicine is used to lower blood pressure.

It is very important that you take this medicine as your doctor has prescribed and that you do not miss any doses. Hypertension (high blood pressure) is a longterm disease and it may be necessary for you to take the drug for a long time in spite of the fact that you feel better. Do not go without the medicine between prescription refills.

If this medicine causes dizziness, you should be careful going up and down stairs and you should not change positions too rapidly. Get out of bed slowly in the morning and dangle your feet over the edge of the bed for a few minutes before standing up. Sit down or lie down at the first sign of dizziness. Tell your doctor you have been dizzy.

In some people, this drug may cause blurred vision. Do not drive a car or operate dangerous machinery or do jobs that require you to be alert until you know how you are going to react to the drug.

Some non-prescription drugs, especially cough and cold remedies, may aggravate your condition. Read the label of the product you select to see if there is a warning. If there is, check with your doctor or pharmacist before using it.

Call your doctor if you develop weight gain and swelling of the ankles, fainting, "ringing" or "buzzing" in the ears or a skin rash.

Metronidazole

Common Trade Names
Flagyl

This medicine is used to treat certain types of infections.

Take the tablets with food or milk.

In some people, this drug may cause dizziness. Do not drive a car or operate machinery or do jobs that require you to be alert until you know how you are going to react to the drug. Sit down or lie down if you become dizzy.

Do not drink alcoholic beverages while taking this medicine because the combination may cause headache, flushing or an upset stomach.

This medicine may cause your urine to turn darker in color. This is not an unusual effect.

It is important to take **all** of the doses that your doctor has prescribed for you. Do not stop taking it earlier than your doctor has recommended in spite of the fact that you may feel better. Otherwise the infection may return.

Call your doctor if you develop a skin rash or a furry tongue.

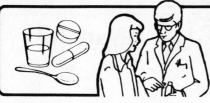

Miconazole

Common Trade Names:
Monistat 7 Vaginal Cream

 This drug is used to treat certain types of fungal infections of the vagina.

Instructions For Use:

● Remove cap from tube of medicine and screw applicator to tube.

● Squeeze the tube and fill the applicator until the plunger is fully extended. If your doctor has prescribed a smaller dose, fill the applicator to the level he has indicated.

● Unscrew the applicator by the cylinder.

● Lie comfortably on your back and gently insert the applicator in the vagina as far as it will comfortably go.

● Press the plunger gently to deposit the drug.

● While keeping the plunger depressed, remove the applicator from the vaginal canal.

● After **each** use, take the applicator apart and wash with soap and warm water. Rinse thoroughly.

● Reassemble. Place the cap on end of the plunger.

During treatment, your doctor may recommend that you do not have sexual intercourse or that your your partner uses a condom.

 Call your doctor if the condition for which this drug is being used continues or becomes worse or if the cream causes a constant irritation such as burning or itching.

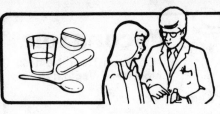

Nadolol

Common Trade Name:
Corgard

This medicine is used to treat a type of chest pain called angina and it is also used to lower blood pressure.

It is very important that you take this medicine as your doctor has directed and that you do not miss any doses. It may be necessary for you to take the drug for a long time in spite of the fact that you feel better. Do not go without medicine between prescription refills.

Take the medicine with food or a glass of water.

In some people, this drug may cause dizziness or drowsiness. Do not drive a car or operate dangerous machinery or do jobs that require you to be alert until you know how you are going to react to this drug. Sit or lie down at the first sign of dizziness.

It is important that you obtain the advice of your doctor before taking cough, cold, or sinus products, asthma or allergy products, diet or weight reducing medicines.

Call your doctor if you develop a skin rash, shortness of breath, fever, sore throat, mouth sores, easy bruising, swelling of the hands or feet, sudden weight gain.

Do not stop taking this medicine suddenly without the approval of your doctor.

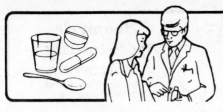

Naproxen

Common Trade Names:
Naprosyn

This medicine is used to help relieve pain, redness and swelling in certain kinds of arthritis and other medical conditions.

The full effect of this medicine will not be noticed immediately but may take from a few days to 3 weeks.

This drug may be taken with food if it upsets your stomach. Call your doctor if you continue to have stomach upset.

In some people, this drug may cause dizziness or drowsiness. Do not drive a car or operate dangerous machinery or do jobs that require you to be alert until you know how you are going to react to this drug.

If you become dizzy, you should be careful going up and down stairs. Sit or lie down at the first sign of dizziness.

Call your doctor if you develop a skin rash, "ringing" or "buzzing" in the ears, black stools or severe stomach pain, swelling of the ankles or blurred vision.

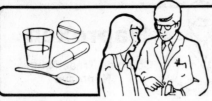

Neomycin-Hydrocortisone-Polymyxin
Common Trade Names:
Cortisporin Otic

 ## This drug is used to treat certain types of ear infections.

If possible, have someone else administer the eardrops for you.

Instructions For Use:

● Warm the drops to body temperature by holding the bottle in your hands for a few minutes. Do NOT heat the drops in hot water.

● If you were prescribed the SUSPENSION, shake the bottle well.

● The person administering the drops should wash his hands with soap and water.

● The eardrops must be kept clean. Do not touch the dropper against the ear or anything else.

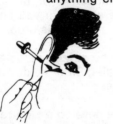

● Tilt your head or lie on your side so that the ear to be treated is facing up.

● In adults, hold the earlobe up and back. In children, hold the earlobe down and back.

● Place the prescribed number of drops of medicine into the ear. Do not insert the dropper into the ear as it may cause injury.

● Remain in the same position for a short time (5 minutes) after you have administered the eardrops.

● Dry the earlobe if there are any drops on it.

Call your doctor if the ear infection becomes worse or lasts for more than 7 days or if the ear becomes swollen, itchy, red or scaly.

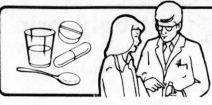

Nitrofurantoin

Common Trade Names:
Furadantin, Macrodantin

This medicine is used to treat certain kinds of infections of the bladder and kidneys.

Take this medicine with food or a full glass of milk.

Try to drink at least eight 8-ounce glasses of water or other fluids a day unless otherwise directed.

If you were prescribed the liquid medicine, shake the bottle well each time you use it so that you can measure an accurate dose.

This medicine may cause the urine to turn brown. This is not an unusual effect and you should not be concerned.

It is important to take **all** of this medicine plus any refills that your doctor told you to take. Do not stop taking it earlier than your doctor has recommended in spite of the fact that you may feel better. Otherwise the infection may return.

Call your doctor if you develop a skin rash, fever or chills, troublesome nausea or diarrhea, numbness in the fingers and toes or difficulty in breathing.

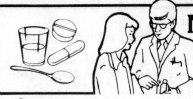

Nitroglycerin

Common Trade Names:
Nitrostat

 This medicine is used to help relieve a type of chest pain called angina.

Carry this medicine with you all the time.

 Keep the tablets in the container supplied by your pharmacist and keep the container tightly closed. This will help keep the tablets fresh.

 This medicine should be used at the first sign of an attack of angina. Sit down or lie down as soon as you feel an attack of angina coming on.

 Do not swallow the tablet but instead place it under the tongue until it is completely dissolved. Do not swallow until the drug is dissolved and do not rinse the mouth for a few minutes.

Take only fresh tablets. If your tablets are more than 1 year old or if they do not produce a tingling or burning sensation when you place them under your tongue, call your doctor or pharmacist to obtain a new supply.

 The first few doses of this medicine may cause dizziness, headache or flushing of the face. This is normal and will disappear after you have taken the drug a few times. Sit down or lie down until these effects pass. Get up slowly from a sitting or lying position.

 Do not drink alcohol too soon after taking this medicine as it may cause an unpleasant effect.

Some non-prescription drugs, especially cough and cold remedies, may aggravate your condition. Read the label of the product you select to see if there is a warning. If there is, check with your doctor or pharmacist before using it.

Call your doctor if you develop blurred vision, a dry mouth or if your chest pain is not relieved after you have taken the number of tablets your doctor has prescribed for an attack.

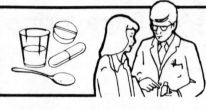

Oxazepam

Common Trade Names:
Serax

This medicine is used to help relieve anxiety and tension and to treat some conditions of the nerves.

In some people, this drug may cause dizziness or drowsiness. Do not drive a car or operate dangerous machinery or do jobs that require you to be alert until you know how you are going to react to this drug.

If you become dizzy, you should be careful going up and down stairs. Sit or lie down at the first sign of dizziness.

Do not drink alcoholic beverages while taking this drug.

It is important that you obtain the advice of your doctor before taking pain relievers, non-prescription drugs, sleeping pills or tranquilizers while you are taking this drug.

Do not take any more of this drug than your doctor has prescribed and do not stop taking this medicine without the approval of your doctor.

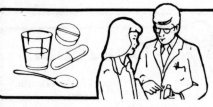

Papaverine

Common Trade Names:
Pavabid

This medicine is used in certain types of conditions to help improve blood flow to cells of the body.

In some people, this drug may cause dizziness or drowsiness. Do not drive a car or operate dangerous machinery or do jobs that require you to be alert until you know how you are going to react to this drug.

If you become dizzy, you should be careful going up and down stairs. Sit or lie down at the first sign of dizziness.

Call your doctor if you develop eye pain, blurred vision, dark-colored urine, yellow color of the skin or eyes.

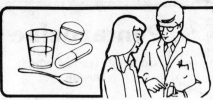

Penicillin VK
Pen-Vee K, V-Cillin K
Penicillin G
Pentids

 This medicine is an antibiotic used to treat certain types of infections.

 It is best to take this medicine on an empty stomach 1 hour before (or 2 hours after) food unless otherwise directed. Take it at the proper time even if you skip a meal.

For Liquid Medicines:

 Store the bottle of medicine in a refrigerator but do not freeze.

Each time you use it, shake the bottle well so that you can measure an accurate dose.

 If a dropper is used to measure the dose and you do not fully understand how to use it, check with your pharmacist.

If there is a discard date on the bottle, throw away any unused medicine after that date. Do not take or save old medicine. Call your pharmacist if you are not sure of the discard date.

 It is important to take **all** of this medicine plus any refills that your doctor told you to take. Do not stop taking this medicine earlier than your doctor has recommended in spite of the fact that you may feel better. Otherwise, the infection may return.

 Contact your doctor should you develop a skin rash, fever, or chills that you did not have before taking the drug.

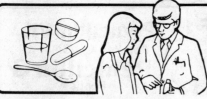

Pentazocine

Common Trade Names:
Talwin

 This medicine is used to help relieve pain.

 Do not take this medicine more often or longer than your doctor has prescribed.

 In some people, this drug may cause dizziness or drowsiness. Do not drive a car or operate dangerous machinery or do jobs that require you to be alert until you know how you are going to react to this drug.

 If you become dizzy, you should be careful going up and down stairs. Sit or lie down at the first sign of dizziness.

 Do not drink alcoholic beverages while taking this drug.

 It is important that you obtain the advice of your doctor before taking other pain relievers, non-prescription drugs, sleeping pills or tranquilizers while you are taking this drug.

Do not stop taking this drug suddenly without the approval of your doctor.

 Call your doctor if you develop "ringing" or "buzzing" in the ears, difficulty in breathing, a change in your mood or depression.

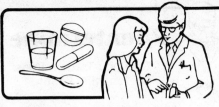

Phenobarbital

Common Trade Names:
Luminal

 This medicine has many uses and the reason it was prescribed depends upon your condition. Check with your doctor if you do not fully understand why you are taking it.

 In some people, this drug may cause dizziness or drowsiness. Do not drive a car or operate dangerous machinery or do jobs that require you to be alert until you know how you are going to react to this drug.

 If you become dizzy, you should be careful going up and down stairs. Sit or lie down at the first sign of dizziness.

 Do not drink alcoholic beverages while taking this drug.

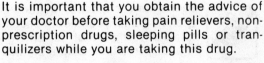 It is important that you obtain the advice of your doctor before taking pain relievers, non-prescription drugs, sleeping pills or tranquilizers while you are taking this drug.

 Do not take any more of this drug than your doctor has prescribed and do not stop taking it suddenly without first asking your doctor.

 If you are taking this medicine to help you sleep, go to bed after you have taken it. Do not smoke in bed after taking the medicine and do not store this medicine at your bedside.

 Call your doctor if you develop bothersome sleepiness during the day, nightmares, staggering or unusual nervousness.

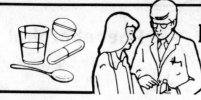

Phentermine

Common Trade Names:
Ionamin, Fastin

 This medicine is used to decrease the appetite in weight reduction programs.

It is important that you follow the diet prescribed by your doctor.

 In some people, this drug may cause dizziness. Do not drive a car or operate dangerous machinery or do jobs that require you to be alert until you know how you are going to react to this drug.

 If you become dizzy, you should be careful going up and down stairs. Sit or lie down at the first sign of dizziness.

 Suck a hard sour candy (sugarless), ice chips or chew gum if your mouth becomes dry. It is especially important to brush your teeth regularly if you develop a dry mouth.

 Do not take any more of this drug than your doctor has prescribed and do not stop taking this medicine suddenly without the approval of your doctor.

 Call your doctor if you develop fast heart rate, or a change in your mood.

Phenylbutazone Oxyphenbutazone

Common Trade Names:
**Azolid A,
Butazolidin Alka**

Common Trade Names
Oxalid, Tandearil

This medicine is used to reduce pain, redness and swelling in certain kinds of arthritis and other medical conditions.

Take this medicine with food or a glass of milk.

Do not use this medicine more often or longer than recommended by your doctor. If you do not feel better after 1 week, call your doctor.

Do not take antacids containing large amounts of sodium while taking this medicine. Check with your pharmacist.

In some people, this drug may cause blurred vision or drowsiness . Do not drive a car or operate dangerous machinery or do jobs that require you to be alert until you know how you are going to react to this drug.

Call your doctor immediately if you develop a skin rash, sore throat, chills or fever, mouth sores, black stools or stomach pain, vomiting, unusual weight gain or swelling of the ankles or face.

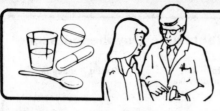

Phenytoin

Common Trade Names:
Dilantin

This medicine is used to help control convulsions or seizures.

Take this medicine with food if it upsets your stomach. Call your doctor if you continue to have stomach upset.

If you were prescribed the liquid medicine, shake the bottle just before using so that you can measure an accurate dose.

It is very important that you take this drug as your doctor has prescribed and that you do not miss any doses. Take this medicine at the same time every day and do not go without this medicine between prescription refills.

Do not stop taking this medicine suddenly without the approval of your doctor.

In some people this drug may cause dizziness or drowsiness. Do not drive a car or operate dangerous machinery or do jobs that require you to be alert until you know how you are going to react to this drug. If you become dizzy, you should be careful going up and down stairs. Sit or lie down at the first sign of dizziness.

Do not drink alcoholic beverages while taking this drug.

It is important that you obtain the advice of your doctor before taking pain relievers, nonprescription drugs, sleeping pills or tranquilizers while you are taking this drug.

While taking this medicine, brush your teeth and gums regularly. The next time you visit your dentist, tell him you are taking this medicine. Call your doctor if your gums become red or swollen.

 Call your doctor if you develop a skin rash, sore throat, fever, mouth sores, persistent headache, slurred speech, joint pain, swollen glands or difficulty in walking.

 Carry a card in your wallet or wear a bracelet stating that you are taking this drug.

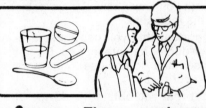

Pilocarpine

Common Trade Names
Isopto-Carpine, Pilocar

 These eyedrops are used to help relieve the symptoms of glaucoma.

If necessary, have someone else administer the eyedrops for you.

Instruction For Use:

● The person administering the eyedrops should wash his hands with soap and water.

● The eyedrops and the container must be kept clean. Do not touch the dropper against the face or anything else.

● Lie down or tilt your head backward and look at the ceiling.

● Gently pull down the lower lid of your eye to form a pouch.

Pilocarpine Continued

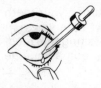

● Hold the dropper in your other hand and approach the eye from the side. Place the dropper as close to the eye as possible without touching it.

● Place the prescribed number of drops into the pouch of the eye.

● Close your eyes. Do not rub them.

● Apply gentle pressure for a minute with your fingers to both sides of the bridge of the nose to prevent the eyedrops from being drained from the eye.

● Blot excess solution around the eye with a tissue.

● Replace top on bottle.

In some people, this drug makes it more difficult for patients to see well, especially at night. Do not drive a car or operate dangerous machinery until you know how you are going to react to this medicine.

It is very important that you use these eyedrops as your doctor has prescribed. Do not miss any doses and do not use them more often than prescribed.

It is important that you obtain the advice of your doctor before taking other medicines and nonprescription drugs such as cold medicines.

Call your doctor if you develop unusual sweating, nausea, fainting or if the eyedrops cause stinging or swelling of the eyes.

Polymyxin-Neomycin-Bacitracin

Common Trade Names:
Neosporin Ophthalmic

This drug is used to treat certain types of eye infections.

If possible, have someone else administer the eye drops for you.

Instructions For Use:

If you were prescribed the EYEDROPS:

• The person administering the eyedrops should wash his hands with soap and water.

• The eyedrops must be kept clean. Do not touch the dropper against the face or anything else.

• Lie down or tilt your head backward and look at the ceiling.

• Gently pull down the lower lid of your eye to form a pouch.

• Hold the dropper in your other hand and approach the eye from the side. Place the dropper as close to the eye as possible without touching it.

• Place the prescribed number of drops into the pouch of the eye.

• Close your eyes. Do not rub them.

• Apply gentle pressure for a minute with your fingers to the bridge of the nose to prevent the eyedrops from being drained from the eye.

• Blot excess solution around the eye with a tissue.

If you were prescribed EYE OINTMENT:

• The person administering the eye ointment should wash his hands with soap and water.

• The eye ointment must be kept clean. Do not touch the tube against the face or anything else.

• Lie down or tilt your head backward and look at the ceiling.

● Gently pull down the lower lid of your eye to form a pouch.

● Hold the tube in your other hand and place the tube as close as possible to the eye without touching it.

● Squeeze the prescribed amount of ointment from the tube along the pouch.

● Close your eyes. Do not rub them.

● Wipe off any excess ointment around the eye with a tissue.

Vision may be blurred for a few minutes after applying the ointment. Do not drive a car or operate dangerous machinery or do jobs that require you to be alert until your vision has cleared.

Call your doctor if the eye infection becomes worse or has not improved within 2 or 3 days.

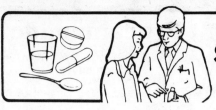

Potassium Supplement

Common Trade Names:
K-Lyte, Slow-K
Potassium Chloride

This medicine is a potassium supplement which is used by people who have certain disease conditions or who are taking prescription medicines that can cause the body to be low in potassium.

If you were prescribed K-LYTE, dissolve the medicine in cold water. Your pharmacist will tell you how much water to use. Let any bubbles disappear before drinking the solution. Sip the medicine slowly over a 5-10 minute period.

If you were prescribed SLOW-K, swallow the tablets whole with a full glass of water. Do not crush, chew or break them into pieces, and do not suck the tablets.

If you were prescribed POTASSIUM CHLORIDE SOLUTION, mix it with a glass of water or fruit juice before taking.

This drug may be taken at the same time as food if it upsets your stomach.

Call your doctor if you develop sharp stomach pain, black stools, a feeling of weakness or heaviness in the legs or a numbness of the hands and feet.

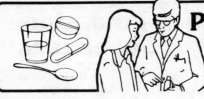

Procainamide

Common Trade Names
Pronestyl

This medicine is used to help make the heart beat at a normal rate.

It is very important that you take this medicine as your doctor has prescribed and that you do not miss any doses. Take this medicine at the same times everyday and do not go without the drug between prescription refills.

Some non-prescription drugs, especially cough and cold remedies, may aggravate your condition. Read the label of the product you select to see if there is a warning. If there is, check with your doctor or pharmacist before using it.

Call your doctor if you develop a sore throat, fever, mouth or gum sores, symptoms of a cold, joint pain or a skin rash.

Store in a cool, dry place. Do not store the medicine in a moist place such as the bathroom medicine cabinet or refrigerator.

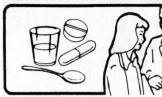

Prochlorperazine

Common Trade Names:
Compazine

This medicine is used to help relieve the symptoms of anxiety, tension and certain types of emotional problems. It is also used to control nausea and vomiting.

If you were prescribed COMPAZINE SPANSULES, swallow the capsules whole. Do not crush, chew or mash the contents.

If you were prescribed **SUPPOSITORIES:**

1. Remove the wrapper from the suppository.

2. Lie on your side and raise your knee to your chest.

3. Insert the suppository with the tapered (pointed) end first into the rectum. Hold the suppository in place for a few minutes.

4. Try to avoid having a bowel movement for at least one hour so that the drug can be absorbed.

In some people, this drug may cause dizziness or drowsiness. Do not drive a car or operate dangerous machinery or do jobs that require you to be alert until you know how you are going to react to this drug.

If this medicine causes dizziness, you should be careful going up and down stairs and should not change positions too rapidly. Get out of bed slowly in the morning and dangle your feet over the edge of the bed for a few minutes before standing up. Sit or lie down at the first sign of dizziness.

Do not drink alcoholic beverages while taking this drug.

It is important that you obtain the advice of your doctor before taking pain relievers, non-prescription drugs, sleeping pills or tranquilizers while you are taking this drug.

This medicine makes some people more sensitive to sunlight or sunlamps. If your skin becomes more sensitive to sunlight, tell your doctor and try to stay out of direct sunlight. While in the sun, wear protective clothing and sunglasses. You may wish to ask your pharmacist about suitable sunscreen products. Call your doctor if you become sunburned.

Suck a hard sour candy (sugarless), ice chips or chew gum if your mouth becomes dry. It is especially important to brush your teeth regularly if you develop a dry mouth.

Do not stop taking this medicine without the approval of your doctor.

Call your doctor if you develop a sore throat, fever, mouth sores, skin rash, changes in eyesight, dizziness, dark-colored urine, a yellow color in the eyes or skin, or unusual movements of the face, tongue or arms.

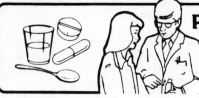

Prochlorperazine-Isopropamide

Common Trade Names:
Combid

This medicine is used to help relax the muscles in certain types of stomach and bowel conditions.

COMBID SPANSULES must be swallowed whole. Do not crush, chew or mash the contents.

In some people, this drug may cause dizziness or drowsiness. Do not drive a car or operate dangerous machinery or do jobs that require you to be alert until you know how you are going to react to this drug.

If this medicine causes dizziness, you should be careful going up and down stairs and you should not change positions too rapidly. Get out of bed slowly in the morning and dangle your feet over the edge of the bed for a few minutes before standing up. Sit or lie down at the first sign of dizziness. Tell your doctor you have been dizzy.

Do not drink alcoholic beverages while taking this drug.

It is important that you obtain the advice of your doctor before taking pain relievers, non-prescription drugs, sleeping pills or tranquilizers while you are taking this drug.

This medicine makes some people more sensitive to sunlight or sunlamps. If your skin becomes more sensitive to sunlight, tell your doctor and try to stay out of direct sunlight. While in the sun, wear protective clothing and sunglasses. You may wish to ask your pharmacist about suitable sunscreen products. Call your doctor if you become sunburned.

Suck a hard sour candy (sugarless), ice chips or chew gum if your mouth becomes dry. It is especially important to brush your teeth regularly if you develop a dry mouth.

Call your doctor if you develop a sore throat, fever, mouth sores, skin rash, changes in eyesight, dark-colored urine, a yellow color in the eyes or skin or unusual movements of the face, tongue or arms.

Promethazine-APC
Synalgos

Promethazine-APC-Codeine
Synalgos-DC

This medicine is used to help relieve pain.

Do not take this medicine more often or longer than your doctor has prescribed.

In some people, this drug may cause dizziness or drowsiness. Do not drive a car or operate dangerous machinery or do jobs that require you to be alert until you know how you are going to react to this drug.

If you become dizzy, you should be careful going up and down stairs. Sit or lie down at the first sign of dizziness.

Do not drink alcoholic beverages while taking this drug.

It is important that you obtain the advice of your doctor before taking other pain relievers, non-prescription drugs, sleeping pills or tranquilizers while you are taking this drug.

This medicine makes some people more sensitive to sunlight or sunlamps. If your skin becomes more sensitive to sunlight, tell your doctor and try to stay out of direct sunlight. While in the sun, wear protective clothing and sunglasses. You may wish to ask your pharmacist about suitable sunscreen products. Call your doctor if you become sunburned.

Call your doctor if you develop a sore throat, fever or mouth sores.

Promethazine-Expectorant
Phenergan Expectorant

Promethazine-Expectorant-Phenylephrine
Phenergan VC Expectorant

Promethazine-Expectorant-Codeine
Phenergan Expectorant/Codeine

Promethazine-Expectorant-Phenylephrine-Codeine
Phenergan VC Expectorant/Codeine

This medicine is used to help relieve the symptoms of coughs and colds and certain types of allergic conditions.

In some people, this drug may cause dizziness or drowsiness. Do not drive a car or operate dangerous machinery or do jobs that require you to be alert until you know how you are going to react to this drug.

If you become dizzy, you should be careful going up and down stairs. Sit or lie down at the first sign of dizziness.

Do not drink alcoholic beverages while taking this drug.

This medicine makes some people more sensitive to sunlight or sunlamps. If your skin becomes more sensitive to sunlight, tell your doctor and try to stay out of direct sunlight. While in the sun, wear protective clothing and sunglasses. You may wish to ask your pharmacist about suitable sunscreen products. Call your doctor if you become sunburned.

It is important that you obtain the advice of your doctor before taking pain relievers, non-prescription drugs, sleeping pills or tranquilizers while you are taking this drug.

Do not use this medicine more often or longer than recommended by your doctor.

Call your doctor if you develop a sore throat, fever or mouth sores.

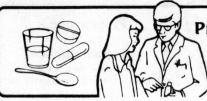

Propoxyphene-APC

Common Trade Names:
**Darvon Compound,
Darvon Compound-65**

This medicine is used to help relieve pain.

Do not take this medicine more often or longer than prescribed by your doctor.

It is best to take this medicine with a glass of water or food to help prevent stomach upset. Call your doctor if you continue to have stomach upset.

In some people this drug may cause drowsiness or dizziness. Do not drive a car or operate dangerous machinery or do jobs that require you to be alert until you know how you are going to react to this drug. If you become dizzy, you should be careful going up and down stairs. Sit or lie down at the first sign of dizziness.

Do not drink alcoholic beverages while taking this drug.

It is important that you obtain the advice of your doctor before taking other pain relievers, non-prescription drugs, sleeping pills or tranquilizers while you are taking this drug.

Call your doctor if you develop "ringing" or "buzzing" in the ears or difficulty hearing, black stools, fever, sweating, wheezing or unusual fatigue or nervousness.

Do not take or save old medicine. Throw away this medicine if it smells like vinegar.

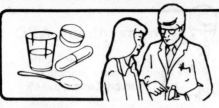

Propoxyphene Napsylate-Acetaminophen

Common Trade Names:
Darvocet-N 100, Darvocet-N 50

This medicine is used to help relieve pain.

Take this medicine with food or milk.

In some people this drug may cause dizziness or drowsiness. Do not drive a car or operate dangerous machinery or do jobs that require you to be alert until you know how you are going to react to this drug.

If you become dizzy, you should be careful going up and down stairs. Sit or lie down at the first sign of dizziness.

Do not drink alcoholic beverages while taking this drug.

It is important that you obtain the advice of your doctor before taking other pain relievers, nonprescription drugs, sleeping pills or tranquilizers while you are taking this drug.

Do not take this medicine more often or longer than your doctor has prescribed.

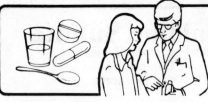

Propranolol

Common Trade Names:
Inderal

This medicine has many uses and the reason it was prescribed depends upon your condition. It is usually used to keep the heart beat slow and steady or to treat high blood pressure. Make sure you understand why you are taking it.

Depending upon your doctor's instructions, this medicine can be taken with a glass of water before or after meals **or** on an empty stomach (1 hour before or 2 hours after meals). It is important to always take it in the same way each day.

In some people this drug may cause drowsiness or dizziness. Do not drive a car or operate dangerous machinery or do jobs that require you to be alert until you know how you are going to react to this drug. If you become dizzy, you should be careful going up and down stairs. Sit or lie down at the first sign of dizziness.

Some non-prescription drugs, especially cough and cold remedies, may aggravate your condition. Read the label of the product you select to see if there is a warning. If there is, check with your doctor or pharmacist before using it.

It is recommended that patients receiving this drug should stop smoking.

Call your doctor if you develop a skin rash or shortness of breath.

Do not stop taking this medicine suddenly without the approval of your doctor.

Quinidine Sulfate
Common Trade Names:
**Quinora,
Quinidex Extentabs**

This medicine is used to make the heart beat strong and steady.

It is very important that you take this medicine as your doctor has directed and that you do not miss any doses. Take this medicine at the same time every day and do not go without this medicine between prescription refills.

The medicine may be taken with food if it upsets your stomach.

If you were prescribed QUINIDEX EXTENTABS, swallow the tablets whole. Do not crush, chew or break them into pieces.

Some non-prescription drugs, especially cough and cold remedies, may aggravate your condition. Read the label of the product you select to see if there is a warning. If there is, check with your doctor or pharmacist before using it.

Call your doctor if you develop "ringing" or "buzzing" in the ears, blurred vision, dizziness, a skin rash, fever, severe headaches, vomiting or troublesome diarrhea.

Reserpine Hydralazine-Hydrochlorothiazide

Common Trade Names:
Ser-Ap-Es

This medicine is used to lower blood pressure.

It is very important that you take this medicine as your doctor has directed and that you do not miss any doses. Hypertension (high blood pressure) is a longterm disease and it may be necessary for you to take the drug for a long time in spite of the fact that you feel better. Do not go without medicine between prescription refills.

Take this medicine with food or milk.

This medicine normally causes your body to lose potassium. The body has warning signs to let you know if too much potassium is being lost. Call your doctor if you become unusually thirsty or if you develop leg cramps or muscle weakness, fatigue, vomiting or confusion. Your doctor may prescribe some medicine to replace the potassium or he may tell you to eat foods which contain a lot of potassium (for example, orange juice, bananas, dates, raisins).

This medicine may make some people more sensitive to sunlight and sunlamps. If your skin becomes more sensitive to sunlight, tell your doctor and try to stay out of direct sunlight. While in the sun, wear protective clothing and sunglasses. You may wish to ask your pharmacist about suitable sunscreen products. Call your doctor if you become sunburned.

Headaches may occur during the first few days and then will usually disappear within the first week. If they continue, call your doctor.

Do not drink alcoholic beverages while taking this drug because the combination may cause dizziness and fainting.

If this medicine causes dizziness, you should be careful going up and down stairs and you should not change positions too rapidly. Get out of bed slowly in the morning and dangle your feet over the edge of the bed for a few minutes before standing up. Sit down or lie down at the first sign of dizziness. Tell your doctor that you have been dizzy. Do not drive a car or operate dangerous machinery if you are dizzy.

This medicine may cause nasal stuffiness. If it becomes bothersome, ask your doctor or pharmacist to recommend a nasal decongestant.

Call your doctor if you develop a sore throat, fever, skin rash, sharp joint pain, stomach pain, or if you develop nightmares or become depressed.

Reserpine-	**Reserpine-**
Hydrochlorothiazide	**Chlorothiazide**
Hydropres	Diupres
Reserpine-	**Reserpine-**
Hydroflumethiazide	**Chlorthalidone**
Salutensin	Regroton, Demi-Regroton

 This medicine is used to lower blood pressure.

 It is very important that you take this medicine as your doctor has directed and that you do not miss any doses. Hypertension (high blood pressure) is a longterm disease and it may be necessary for you to take the drug for a long time in spite of the fact that you feel better. Do not go without medicine between prescription refills.

Take the medicine with food or milk.

 This medicine normally causes your body to lose potassium. The body has warning signs to let you know if too much potassium is being lost. Call your doctor if you become unusually thirsty, or if you develop leg cramps or muscle weakness, fatigue, vomiting or confusion. Your doctor may prescribe some medicine to replace the potassium or he may tell you to eat foods which contain a lot of potassium (for example, orange juice, bananas, dates, raisins).

 This medicine makes some people more sensitive to sunlight and sunlamps. If your skin becomes more sensitive to sunlight, tell your doctor and try to stay out of direct sunlight. While in the sun, wear protective clothing and sunglasses. You may wish to ask your pharmacist about suitable sunscreen products. Call your doctor if you become sunburned.

If this medicine causes dizziness, you should be careful going up and down stairs and you should not change positions too rapidly. Get out of bed slowly in the morning and dangle your feet over the edge of the bed for a few minutes before standing up. Sit down or lie down at the first sign of dizziness. Tell your doctor you have been dizzy. Do not drive a car or operate dangerous machinery if you are dizzy.

This medicine may cause nasal stuffiness. If it becomes bothersome, ask your doctor or pharmacist to recommend a nasal decongestant.

Call your doctor if you develop a sore throat, fever, skin rash, sharp joint pain or if you develop nightmares or become depressed.

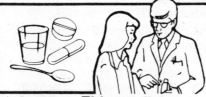

Spironolactone-
Hydrochlorothiazide
Common Trade Names:
Aldactazide

This medicine is used to help rid the body of excess fluids, decrease swelling and to treat high blood pressure.

It is very important that you take the medicine as your doctor has directed. Try to remember to take all your doses.

Take this medicine at the same time each day. When you first start taking this medicine, you will probably urinate (pass your water) more often and in larger amounts than usual. Therefore, do not initially take it at bedtime or you may have to get up during the night to go to the bathroom.

Take the drug with or after food.

This medicine may make some people more sensitive to sunlight and sunlamps. If your skin becomes more sensitive to sunlight, tell your doctor and try to stay out of direct sunlight. While in the sun, wear protective clothing and sunglasses. You may wish to ask your pharmacist about suitable sunscreen products. Call your doctor if you become sunburned.

If this medicine causes dizziness, you should be careful going up and down stairs and you should not change positions too rapidly. Get out of bed slowly in the morning and dangle your feet over the edge of the bed for a few minutes before standing up. Sit down or lie down at the first sign of dizziness.

Call your doctor and tell him you have been dizzy. Be careful drinking alcoholic beverages while taking this medicine because it can make this dizziness worse. Do not drive a car or operate dangerous machinery if you are dizzy.

Call your doctor if you develop sharp joint pain, sore throat, fever, skin rash, weakness, dizziness or (in men) swelling and tenderness of the breasts.

Sulfamethoxazole
Gantanol, Gantanol DS

Sulfisoxazole
Gantrisin

Sulfamethoxazole-Trimethoprim
Bactrim, Bactrim DS, Septra, Septra DS

Sulfisoxazole-Phenazopyridine
Azo Gantrisin

 This medicine is an antibiotic used to treat certain types of infections.

 Take the medicine with a full glass of water and try to drink at least eight 8-ounce glasses of water or other fluids a day unless otherwise directed.

 If you were prescribed a liquid SUSPENSION, shake the bottle well each time you use it so that you can measure an accurate dose.

 This medicine makes some people more sensitive to sunlight or sunlamps. If your skin becomes more sensitive to sunlight, tell your doctor and try to stay out of direct sunlight. While in the sun, wear protective clothing and sunglasses. You may wish to ask your pharmacist about suitable sunscreen products. Call your doctor if you become sunburned.

If you were prescribed AZO GANTRISIN, your urine may turn orange-red in color. This is not an unusual effect. Protect your undergarments while you are taking this medicine as your urine could cause staining.

 It is important to take **all** of this medicine plus any refills that your doctor told you to take. Do not stop taking it earlier than your doctor has recommended in spite of the fact that you may feel better. Otherwise, the infection may return.

 Call your doctor if you develop a skin rash, sore throat, fever, mouth sores or dizziness.

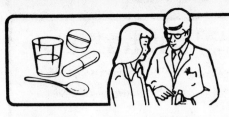

Sulindac

Common Trade Name:
Clinoril

 This medicine is used to help relieve pain, redness, stiffness and swelling in certain kinds of arthritis and other medical conditions.

 Take this medicine with food or a glass of milk or immediately after meals to help prevent stomach upset. If stomach pain persists, contact your doctor.

You may have to take this medicine for 1-2 weeks before you begin to feel its full benefits.

 In some people, this drug may cause dizziness. Do not drive a car or operate dangerous machinery or do jobs that require you to be alert until you know how you are going to react to this drug.

 If you become dizzy, you should be careful going up and down stairs. Sit or lie down at the first sign of dizziness.

 While you are taking this medicine, do not drink alcoholic beverages or take aspirin without the permission of your doctor. It is usually safe to take acetaminophen for the occasional headache. Check with your pharmacist.

 Call your doctor if you develop "ringing" or "buzzing" in the ears, skin rash, swelling of the legs or ankles or a sudden weight gain, stomach pain, red or black stools, changes in your hearing or eyesight or if you become depressed.

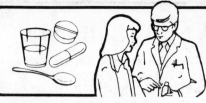

Tetracycline

Common Trade Names:
Achromycin V, Panmycin, Robitet, Sumycin, Tetracyn

This medicine is an antibiotic used to treat certain types of infections and skin conditions.

It is best to take the medicine with a glass of water on an empty stomach at least 1 hour before or 2 hours after drinking milk, or eating cheese, cottage cheese, ice cream or other dairy products. Take it at the proper time even if you skip a meal. If you develop stomach upset after taking the drug, take it with some crackers (not with dairy products). Call your doctor if you continue to have stomach upset.

For Liquid Medicines:

Each time you use it, shake the bottle well so that you can measure an accurate dose.

If there is a discard date on the bottle, throw away any unused medicine after that date. Do not take or save old medicine. Call your pharmacist if you are not sure of the discard date.

If you must take iron products or vitamins containing iron, take them 2 hours before (or 3 hours after) this medicine.

Some antacids can make this medicine less effective if they are taken at the same time. If you must take antacids, they should be taken at least 3 hours after this medicine. If you have any questions, ask your pharmacist.

This medicine may make some people more sensitive to sunlight or sunlamps. If your skin becomes more sensitive to sunlight, tell your doctor and try to stay out of direct sunlight. While in the sun, wear protective clothing and sunglasses. You may wish to ask your pharmacist about suitable sunscreen products. Call your doctor if you become sunburned.

 Call your doctor if you develop a skin rash, sore mouth, troublesome diarrhea (loose bowel movements), or (in women) a vaginal discharge which was not present before you started taking this medicine.

 It is important to take **all** of this medicine plus any refills that your doctor told you to take. Do not stop taking it earlier than your doctor has recommended in spite of the fact that you may feel better. Otherwise, the infection may return.

 If for some reason you cannot take all of the medicine, discard the unused portion by flushing it down the toilet. Do not save this medicine for future use because old tetracycline can cause serious problems.

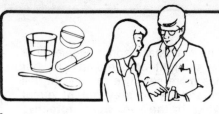

Theophylline-Ephedrine-Hydroxyzine

Common Trade Names:
Marax

This medicine is used to open up the air passages in the lungs and to make it easier to breathe. It is used to treat and control bronchial asthma and bronchospasms.

Take this medicine with some food followed by a glass of water.

In some people, this drug may cause drowsiness. Do not drive a car or operate dangerous machinery or do jobs that require you to be alert until you know how you are going to react to this drug.

Do not drink alcoholic beverages while taking this drug.

It is important that you obtain the advice of your doctor before taking pain relievers, non-prescription drugs, sleeping pills or tranquilizers while you are taking this drug.

Suck a hard sour candy (sugarless), ice chips or chew gum if your mouth becomes dry. It is especially important to brush your teeth regularly if you develop a dry mouth.

Do NOT take this medicine at the same time as a non-prescription drug containing aminophylline or theophylline without the approval of your doctor.

Call your doctor if you develop a sore throat, fever, mouth sores, skin rash or fast heart beats.

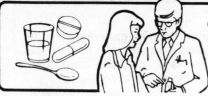

Thioridazine

Common Trade Names:
Mellaril

 This medicine is used to help relieve anxiety and tension and some types of emotional problems.

 If a dropper is used to measure the dose and you do not fully understand how to use it, check with your pharmacist. The liquid medicine can be added to water, fruit juices, soft drinks, coffee or tea just before you take it.

 The full effect of this medicine will not be noticed immediately but may take from a few days to 4 weeks.

 In some people, this drug may cause dizziness or drowsiness. Do not drive a car or operate dangerous machinery or do jobs that require you to be alert until you know how you are going to react to this drug.

 If this medicine causes dizziness, you should be careful going up and down stairs and you should not change positions too rapidly. Get out of bed slowly in the morning and dangle your feet over the edge of the bed for a few minutes before standing. Sit or lie down at the first sign of dizziness. Tell your doctor you have been dizzy.

 Do not drink alcoholic beverages while taking this drug.

It is important that you obtain the advice of your doctor before taking pain relievers, non-prescription drugs, sleeping pills or tranquilizers while you are taking this drug.

Thioridazine Continued

Suck a hard sour candy (sugarless), ice chips or chew gum if your mouth becomes dry. It is especially important to brush your teeth regularly if you develop a dry mouth.

Do not stop taking this medicine suddenly without the approval of your doctor.

This medicine may make some people more sensitive to sunlight and sunlamps. If your skin becomes more sensitive to sunlight, tell your doctor and try to stay out of direct sunlight. While in the sun, wear protective clothing and sunglasses. You may wish to ask your pharmacist about suitable sunscreen products. Call your doctor if you become sunburned.

Call your doctor if you develop a sore throat, fever, mouth sores, dark-colored urine, a yellow color in the eyes or skin, changes in vision, unusual movements of the face, tongue or arms, or difficulty in urinating (passing your water).

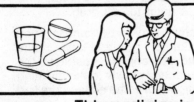

Thyroid Hormone

Common Trade Names:
**Cytomel, Levothroid
Proloid, Synthroid**

This medicine is a hormone which is used to treat certain thyroid disorders.

Take this medicine at the same time every day and do not go without this medicine between prescription refills.

Call your doctor if you develop chest pain, fast heart beat, unusual diarrhea (loose bowel movements), nervousness, excessive sweating, headaches or difficulty sleeping.

Some nonprescription drugs, especially cough and cold remedies, may aggravate your condition. Read the label of the product you select to see if there is a warning. If there is, check with your doctor or pharmacist before using it.

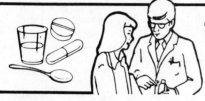

Tolazamide

Common Trade Names
Tolinase

This medicine is used in the treatment of diabetes.

Know the signs of hypoglycemia (low blood sugar). Call your doctor if you develop weakness, sweating or shaking that is not relieved by eating or drinking something sweet.

It is very important that you take this drug as your doctor has prescribed and that you do not miss any doses. Take this medicine at the same time everyday and do not go without this medicine between prescription refills.

Take the drug with food if it upsets your stomach. Call your doctor if you continue to have stomach upset.

It is recommended that you avoid the use of alcoholic beverages because the combination may cause headache, flushing, an upset stomach or hypoglycemia (low blood sugar).

Your doctor or pharmacist can tell you which

nonprescription medicines (for example, cough medicines) are safe for diabetic patients. It is recommended that you do not take drugs containing salicylates (for example, aspirin) because the combination may cause hypoglycemia (low blood sugar).

This medicine makes some people more sensitive to sunlight or sunlamps. If your skin becomes more sensitive to sunlight, tell your doctor and try to stay out of direct sunlight. While in the sun, wear protective clothing and sunglasses. You may wish to ask your pharmacist about suitable sunscreen products. Call your doctor if you become sunburned.

Call your doctor if you develop a sore throat, fever, mouth sores, skin rash, dark-colored urine, light-colored stools or a yellow color in the skin or eyes.

Carry a card in your wallet or wear a bracelet stating that you are a diabetic.

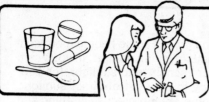

Tolbutamide

Common Trade Names:
Orinase

This medicine is used in the treatment of diabetes.

Know the signs of hypoglycemia (low blood sugar). Call your doctor if you develop weakness, sweating or shaking that is not relieved by eating or drinking something sweet.

It is very important that you take this drug as your doctor has prescribed and that you do not miss any doses. Take this medicine at the same time every day and do not go without this medicine between prescription refills. Follow the diet your doctor has prescribed for you.

Take the drug with food if it upsets your stomach. Call your doctor if you continue to have stomach upset.

It is recommended that you avoid the use of alcoholic beverages because the combination may cause headache, flushing, an upset stomach or hypoglycemia (low blood sugar).

Your doctor or pharmacist can tell you which nonprescription medicines (for example, cough and cold medicines) are safe for diabetic patients. It is recommended that patients do not take drugs containing salicylates (for example, aspirin) because the combination may cause hypoglycemia (low blood sugar).

This medicine makes some people more sensitive to sunlight or sunlamps. If your skin becomes more sensitive to sunlight, tell your doctor and try to stay out of direct sunlight. While in the sun, wear protective clothing and sunglasses. You may wish to ask your pharmacist about suitable sunscreen products. Call your doctor if you become sunburned.

Call your doctor if you develop a sore throat, fever, mouth sores, skin rash, dark-colored urine, light-colored stools or a yellow color in the skin or eyes

Carry a card in your wallet or wear a bracelet stating that you are a diabetic.

Triamicinolone-Neomycin-Gramicidin-Nystatin

Common Trade Names:
Mycolog

This drug is used to treat certain types of skin conditions.

Instructions for use:

1. Cleanse the skin area well with soap and water unless otherwise directed by your doctor. Allow the skin to dry completely or pat dry with a clean towel.

2. Apply the drug to the affected area and rub in lightly. Do not bandage unless directed by your doctor.

Do not use the drug more frequently or in larger quantities than prescribed by your doctor.

Do not apply cosmetics or lotions on top of the drug unless your doctor approves.

Call your doctor if the condition for which this medicine is being used persists or becomes worse, or if it causes a constant irritation such as itching or burning.

For external use only. Keep this drug away from the eyes.

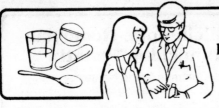

Triamterene
Hydrochlorothiazide

Common Trade Names:
Dyazide

This medicine is used to help rid the body of excess fluids, decrease swelling and to treat high blood pressure.

It is very important that you take the medicine as your doctor has directed. Try to remember to take all your doses.

Take this medicine at the same time each day. When you first start taking this medicine, you will probably urinate (pass your water) more often and in larger amounts than usual. Therefore, do not initially take it at bedtime or you may have to get up during the night to go to the bathroom.

Take the drug with or after food.

This medicine may make some people more sensitive to sunlight and sunlamps. If your skin becomes more sensitive to sunlight, tell your doctor and try to stay out of direct sunlight. While in the sun, wear protective clothing and sunglasses. You may wish to ask your pharmacist about suitable sunscreen products. Call your doctor if you become sunburned.

If this medicine causes dizziness, you should be careful going up and down stairs and you should not change positions too rapidly. Get out of bed slowly in the morning and dangle your feet over the edge of the bed for a few minutes before standing up. Sit down or lie down at the first sign of dizziness. Call your doctor and tell him you have been dizzy. Be careful drinking alcoholic beverages while taking this medicine because it can make this dizziness worse. Do not drive a car or operate dangerous machinery if you are dizzy.

Call your doctor if you develop sharp joint pain, sore throat, fever, skin rash, weakness, or headache.

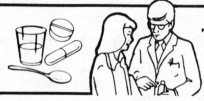

Trifluoperazine

Common Trade Names:
Stelazine

This medicine is used to help relieve the symptoms of anxiety and tension and certain types of emotional problems.

In some people, this drug may cause dizziness or drowsiness. Do not drive a car or operate dangerous machinery or do jobs that require you to be alert until you know how you are going to react to this drug.

If this medicine causes dizziness, you should be careful going up and down stairs and you should not change positions too rapidly. Get out of bed slowly in the morning and dangle your feet over the edge of the bed for a few minutes before standing up. Sit or lie down at the first sign of dizziness. Tell your doctor you have been dizzy.

Do not drink alcoholic beverages while taking this drug.

It is important that you obtain the advice of your doctor before taking pain relievers, non-prescription drugs, sleeping pills or tranquilizers while you are taking this drug.

Suck a hard sour candy (sugarless), ice chips or chew gum if your mouth becomes dry. It is especially important to brush your teeth regularly if you develop a dry mouth.

Do not stop taking this medicine suddenly without the approval of your doctor.

Call your doctor if you develop a sore throat, fever, mouth sores, skin rash, changes in eyesight, dark-colored urine, a yellow color in the eyes or skin, or unusual movements of the face, tongue or arms.

Triprolidine-Pseudoephedrine
Actifed

Triprolidine-Pseudoephedrine-Guaifenesin-Codeine
Actifed-C Expectorant

This medicine is used to help relieve nasal stuffiness and make breathing easier. It is also used for certain types of earaches, allergies and coughs.

This drug may be taken with food or a glass of water or milk if it upsets your stomach.

In some people this drug may cause dizziness or drowsiness. Do not drive a car or operate dangerous machinery or do jobs that require you to be alert until you know how you are going to react to this drug. If you become dizzy, you should be careful going up and down stairs. Sit or lie down at the first sign of dizziness.

Do not drink alcoholic beverages while you are taking this drug.

It is important that you obtain the advice of your doctor before taking pain relievers, non-prescription drugs, sleeping pills or tranquilizers while you are taking this drug.

Suck a hard sour candy (sugarless), ice chips or chew gum if your mouth becomes dry. It is especially important to brush your teeth regularly if you develop a dry mouth.

Do not use this medicine more often or longer than recommended by your doctor.

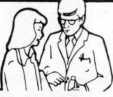

Warfarin

Common Trade Names:
Coumadin

This medicine is used to help prevent harmful blood clots from forming. It is commonly called a "blood thinner".

It is very important that you take this medicine exactly as your doctor has prescribed and that you do not miss any doses. Try to take this medicine at the same time every day. Do not take extra tablets without your doctor's approval.

Regular blood tests are necessary in order for your doctor to prescribe the correct dose for you. Your dose may vary from time to time depending on these tests.

Do not take any other drugs or stop taking any drugs you are presently taking without first consulting your doctor. Do not go without this medicine between prescription refills.

Do not eat large amounts of leafy, green vegetables or change your diet without telling your doctor.

Do not treat yourself with any product containing aspirin or salicylate. This includes many pain killers and antacids. Your pharmacist can tell you which products to avoid.

Know which brand of medicine you are taking and always take the same brand.

If you have a tendency to cut yourself while shaving, you may wish to use an electric razor.

Do not drink alcoholic beverages while you are taking this drug because the combination may cause undesirable side effects.

You may wish to carry an identification card indicating that you are taking this medicine. Always tell your dentist and other doctors who are treating you that you are taking this medicine.

Call your doctor if you miss two doses, or develop any unusual signs of bleeding (for example, bleeding from the nose, mouth or gums after brushing teeth), unusual bruising, red or dark-brown urine or red or black stools.

NONPRESCRIPTION DRUGS
(Ask your pharmacist to approve these drugs before you take them.)

Date	Name of Product

Carry this in your wallet

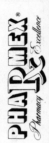

PHARMEX®
Pharmacy Excellence

PERSONAL MEDICATION RECORD

Name: _____
Address: _____

Phone No.: _____
Family Doctor to call in an Emergency:

Name _____ Phone No. _____

ALLERGIES TO DRUGS: _____

Special Medical Problems: _____

133

Date	Prescription Number	Name of Medicine	Directions	Quantity

Name of Pharmacy

Cut along this line.

Carry this in your wallet

PHARMEX®
Pharmacy of Excellence

PERSONAL MEDICATION RECORD

Name: _____
Address: _____
_____

Phone No.: _____
Family Doctor to call in an Emergency:

Name _____ Phone No.

ALLERGIES TO DRUGS: _____
_____

Special Medical Problems: _____
_____

© Copyright 1981 ABP/PHARMEX

NONPRESCRIPTION DRUGS
(Ask your pharmacist to approve these drugs before you take them.)

Date	Name of Product

135

Name of Pharmacy

Date	Prescription Number	Name of Medicine	Directions	Quantity

HOW TO ADMINISTER EYE DROPS

- The person administering the eye drops should wash his hands with soap and water.
- The eye drops must be kept clean. Do not touch the dropper against the face or anything else.
- Lie down or tilt your head backward and look at the ceiling.

- Gently pull down the lower lid of your eye to form a pouch.
- Hold the dropper in your other hand and approach the eye from the side. Place the dropper as close to the eye as possible without touching it.
- Place the prescribed number of drops into the pouch of the eye.

- Close your eyes. Do not rub them.
- Apply gentle pressure for a minute with your fingers to the bridge of the nose to prevent the eye drops from being drained from the eye.
- Blot the excess solution around the eye with a tissue.

If necessary, have someone else administer the eye drops for you.

Some eye drops may blur the vision for a few minutes after using them. Do not drive a car or operate dangerous machinery or do jobs that require you to be alert until your vision has cleared.

Call your doctor if the condition for which the eye drops is being used persists or becomes worse or if they cause itching or burning for more than just a few minutes after use. Many eye drops sting for a short time after use.

Keep the eye drop bottle tightly closed when not in use.

HOW TO ADMINISTER EYE OINTMENTS

- The person administering the eye ointment should wash his hands with soap and water.
- The eye ointment must be kept clean. Do not touch the tube against the face or anything else.

  - Lie down or tilt your head backward and look at the ceiling.
  - Gently pull down the lower lid of your eye to form a pouch.
  - Hold the tube in your hand and place the tube as close as possible to the eye without touching it.

- Squeeze the prescribed amount of ointment (Usually ½ inch) from the tube along the pouch.
- Close your eyes. Do not rub them.
- Wipe off any excess ointment around the eye with a tissue.
- Clean the tip of the ointment tube with a tissue.

If necessary, have someone else administer the eye ointment for you.

Vision may be blurred for a few minutes after applying the ointment. Do not drive a car or operate dangerous machinery or do jobs that require you to be alert until your vision has cleared.

Call your doctor if the condition for which the eye ointment is being used persists or becomes worse or if it causes itching or burning for more than just a few minutes after use. Some eye ointments sting for a short time immediately after use.

Keep the eye ointment tube tightly closed when not in use.

138

HOW TO ADMINISTER EAR DROPS

- Warm the ear drops to body temperature by holding the bottle in your hands for a few minutes. Do NOT heat the drops in hot water.
- The person administering the ear drops should wash his hands with soap and water.
- The ear drops must be kept clean. Do not touch the dropper against the ear or anything else.

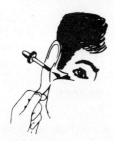

- Tilt your head or lie on your side so that the ear to be treated is facing up.
- In ADULTS, hold the earlobe up and back. In CHILDREN, hold the earlobe down and back.

- Place the prescribed number of drops into the ear. Do not insert the dropper into the ear as it may cause injury.
- Remain in the same position for a short time (5 minutes) after you have administered the drops.
- Dry the earlobe if there are any drops on it.

If necessary, have someone else administer the ear drops for you.

Call your doctor if the condition for which these ear drops is being used persists or becomes worse or if the ear drops cause itching or burning for more than just a few minutes after use.

Do not use the ear drops if they change in color or change in any way since being purchased.

Keep the bottle tightly closed when not in use.

For external use only. Do not swallow.

HOW TO ADMINISTER NOSE DROPS

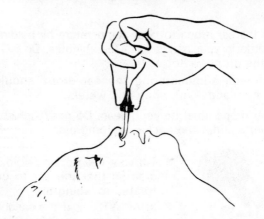

- Blow nose gently before administration of drops.
- Sit in chair and tilt head backward or lie down on bed with head extending over edge of bed or lie down and place a pillow under the shoulders so that the head is tipped backward.
- Insert dropper into nostril about ⅓ inch and drop the prescribed number of drops into the nose.
- Try not to touch the side of the nose with the dropper as it will probably make you sneeze and will contaminate the dropper.
- Remain in the same position for at least 5 minutes.

Do not use this medication for a long period of time or more often than directed.

For external use only.

INDEX

Portions of this book have been reprinted from Smith, D. L., **Medication Guide for Patient Counseling**. Exclusive permission granted by Lea & Febiger, Philadelphia, publisher.